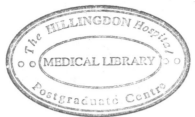
Cardiovascular Monitoring

WITHDRAWN

T

17·00

Cardiovascular Monitoring

Nigel I Jowett

MD, MRCP, MB BS, MRCS, LRCP

Director of Clinical Medicine and Consultant Physician
Pembrokeshire Health Trust, Wales

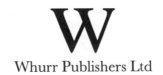

Whurr Publishers Ltd

© 1997 Whurr Publishers Ltd
First published 1997 by
Whurr Publishers Ltd
19b Compton Terrace, London N1 2UN, England

British Library Cataloguing in Publication Data
A catalogue record for this book is available from the
British Library.

ISBN 1 86156 005 2

Printed and bound in the UK by Athenaeum Press Ltd,
Gateshead, Tyne & Wear

Contents

Preface

Those of us in hospital practice are involved in cardiovascular monitoring every working day, whether this is simple recording of the pulse and blood pressure, or complex invasive haemodynamic monitoring in high dependency units. Despite this, observations are often poorly acquired and poorly documented. This is frequently because the reasons for monitoring are poorly understood and the methodology for obtaining good data is poorly taught. Another frequent belief is that monitoring is somehow therapeutic; once the monitor has been connected, the patient is safe and does not need so much attention. Of course, nothing could be further from the truth. The value of such monitoring depends upon somebody watching, understanding what they see, and knowing what to do about any abnormalities. If these cannot be guaranteed, then there is little point in monitoring.

This book is designed to explain the theory and practice of common monitoring techniques. A better understanding should lead to better data collection upon which important therapeutic decisions have to be made, which can only benefit our patients.

Nigel I. Jowett

Dedication

"I am a camera, with its shutter open, quite passive, recording, not thinking"

Christopher Isherwood
"Goodbye to Berlin"

This book is dedicated to those who want to understand

For Alex and Lucy

Chapter 1
Essential Anatomy and Physiology of the Cardiovascular System

The cardiovascular system is a continuous, closed, blood filled circuit equipped with a variable double pump, the heart, which maintains two separate circulations. The *pulmonary circulation* is a low pressure system taking blood to and from the lungs. The *systemic circulation* is a high pressure system conveying blood around the remainder of the body. The systemic circulation contains about 85% of the blood volume, two-thirds of which lies within the veins. The capacitance of these vessels can vary by 2–3 litres in response to veno-dilatation and veno-constriction which maintains an adequate venous return to the heart and helps vary the cardiac output. In contrast, the arteries are very muscular and the arterial lumens are fairly small. Hence, there is not much blood in the arterial system at any one time (about two-thirds of a litre). However, selective vaso-constriction and vaso-dilatation of individual vessels allows the arterial system to regulate the blood supply to the different capillary beds, and thus divert the blood to where it is needed. The typical distribution of the blood volume and cardiac output is shown in Tables 1.1a and 1.1b.

Table 1.1a: Approximate Distribution of the Blood Volume (ml) in a 75 kg Man

	Systemic vessels	Pulmonary vessels
Arteries	640	120
Capillaries	240	140
Vein	3720	240
Heart	200 in each side	

Total blood volume = 5.5 litres

Table 1.1b: Approximate Distribution of the Blood (at Rest) to the Body Organs

	Blood flow (ml/minute)	% Cardiac output
Liver/Gut	1100	20
Kidneys	1100	20
Muscle	1100	20
Brain	825	15
Bone/Fat	825	15
Skin	275	5
Heart	275	5
Cardiac output = 5.5 litres		100%

During vigorous exercise, the cardiac output may increase by a factor of four (to about 20 litres/minute), and the distribution of blood to the organs changes. About 80% of the cardiac output is diverted from the skin, fat, the gut and kidneys to exercising muscles. Cerebral autoregulation ensures that perfusion of the brain is unchanged (still at about 800 ml/minute), but coronary perfusion increases in proportion to the increase in cardiac output, remaining at about 5% of the total.

The Systemic Circulation

The systemic circulation receives oxygenated blood pumped by the left ventricle, through the aorta and into the major arteries. The blood is distributed to the capillary beds by the muscular arterioles. The blood is eventually collected by the venous system and returned to the right atrium. Whilst the blood vessels ensure proper distribution of the blood, it is the capillary beds where the major function of the cardiovascular system takes place. This is the process of metabolic exchange whereby oxygen and nutrients are delivered to the cells and waste products are removed. Tissue perfusion is directly proportional to the rate of blood flow which is ensured by the maintenance of an adequate blood volume and blood pressure.

The Arterial System

Arteries carry blood away from the heart to the major organs and peripheries, and then divide into smaller arterioles. The arterial walls contain large amounts of elastic tissue which are vital in smoothing out the pulsatile blood flow and changing it to a steady, high pressure flow. This is achieved by the arterial walls distending in systole to cushion the initial high pressure wave, and then recoiling in diastole to propel blood forward and maintaining pressure until the next cycle. Hence, by the time the arterioles are reached, there is a steady flow of blood. The arteriolar walls contain richly innervated smooth muscle cells which lie in a state of partial contraction due to continuous sympathetic activity originating in the vasomotor centre in the medulla. This state is referred to as *sympathetic tone*. Changes in activity in the vasomotor centre enable the arterioles to vary the size of their lumens (vaso-constriction or vaso-dilatation) which enables them to divert the blood to the different capillary beds as required.

As the blood moves through the vessels, its progress is slowed both by friction with the vessel walls and its own viscosity. Resistance to arterial blood flow is governed primarily by the arterioles, which are the main resistance vessels. The arteriolar lumen may be narrowed by selective vaso-constriction, spasm or atheromatous deposits. The rate of flow decreases in direct proportion to the fourth power of its diameter (according to Poiseuille's Law). Hence, if the arteriolar lumen is reduced by 50%, the resistance to flow is increased sixteen times.

The average resistance offered by the blood vessels to flow is termed the *systemic vascular resistance* (SVR) or *mean peripheral resistance.*

This is calculated by:

$$\frac{\text{Mean arterial blood pressure} - \text{Central venous pressure}}{\text{Cardiac output}} \quad \text{Units}$$

The Capillary Network

The capillaries are microscopic vessels which connect the arterioles to the venules. They are composed of a single layer of endothelial cells which are selectively permeable to water, electrolytes and nutrients. Permeability can vary in different capillary beds. In the liver and kidney, they are highly permeable whilst elsewhere the capillaries may demonstrate selective permeability, ie. they may be permeable to low molecular weight substances (eg. glucose, ions), but impermeable to high molecular weight plasma proteins.

Since each arteriole feeds many capillaries in parallel, the resistance from the capillary beds is less than the resistance from the arterioles. Muscular vessels at the start of the capillary beds (pre-capillary sphincters) help regulate flow through the capillary bed such that there is active flow in some vessels, but stasis in others. The normal systemic capillary blood volume at rest forms about 6% of the total blood volume (about 300 ml), at an average pressure of between 25–35 mmHg.

The Venous System

The venous system collects the blood from the capillary beds and returns it to the heart. The pulsatile effect of the cardiac cycle is filtered out by the capillary networks, so that venous flow is non-pulsatile. The pressure is low, averaging 5–15 mmHg, but influenced by gravity. In the feet, venous pressure may be as high as 90 mmHg on standing, whilst in the head and neck the pressure may be negative. At the level of the heart, the central venous pressure (CVP) in the right atrium and vena cavae lies between 0–8 mmHg.

Backward flow in the veins is prevented by valves, and forward flow is encouraged by the pressure of blood pushing from behind, and the squeezing effect of surrounding skeletal muscle which helps empty the veins during exercise. The small amount of smooth muscle present in the walls of veins is not able to produce large reductions in the diameter of the vein, but can help regulate venous return by contraction and dilatation to alter the capacitance of the venous system. At rest, 70% of the circulating volume lies in the veins which act as a reservoir to fill the heart at a rate needed to ensure the required cardiac output.

The Pulmonary Circulation

The pulmonary circulation runs in series with the systemic circulation. It receives deoxygenated blood from around the body into the right atrium. This then passes into the right ventricle which propels it into the short main pulmonary trunk, which lies within the pericardial cavity. The pulmonary trunk divides into right and left pulmonary arteries which carry blood to the hila of both lungs. The blood passes through the pulmonary vasculature, and following gaseous exchange in the alveoli, is gathered into four pulmonary veins which deliver the oxygenated blood to the left atrium. Hence in contrast to the systemic circulation, pulmonary arterial blood is therefore deoxygenated and pulmonary venous blood is oxygenated.

The pulmonary circulation differs from the systemic circulation in several ways. In comparison to the systemic circulation, the pulmonary circulation is a low pressure circuit, with a maximum systolic blood pressure one-fifth of the systemic systolic blood pressure. There are no resistance vessels such as arterioles within the circuit, so that flow through the pulmonary capillaries is pulsatile. What resistance exists is caused by the pulmonary capillary network and pulmonary venules. It is referred to as the *pulmonary vascular resistance* (PVR).

There are no valves in the pulmonary veins, which are thin walled and easily distended. This enables a large volume of blood to be held in the pulmonary circulation at any one time (up to a litre), the capacity being higher on inspiration. Because the pulmonary blood pressures are low, gravity affects perfusion of the lungs. Whilst standing, pressure in the vessels at the apices of the lung is low, whilst at the lung bases it is high. On lying down these pressures equilibrate, but will differ between lungs if the subject lies on one side, pressure being higher in the dependent lung. These pressure differences may lead to inequalities of blood and air flow to the lungs (shunting). For example, the apices of the lung will be fully ventilated, but not fully perfused.

The pulmonary vessels are supplied by sympathetic vasoconstrictor fibres. In addition, anoxia and acidaemia will lead to vaso-constriction. Chronic hypoxia leads to chronic vaso-constriction and pulmonary hypertension.

The Heart

The heart is a hollow muscular organ which is located behind the sternum in the middle of the chest, lying two-thirds to the left and one-third to the right. The heart is approximately the size of the subject's clenched fist and weighs about 300 g in the adult male, and 250 g in women. It lies obliquely in the chest, roughly resembling an inverted cone with the base facing upwards, and the apex pointing downwards, forwards and to the left (Figure 1.1). The apex beat marks the outer border of the heart in life, and may be seen pulsating a little below and medial to the left nipple in the 5th intercostal space. This position is variable since tall, thin people tend to have a more vertically placed heart, whereas short, fat individuals have a more horizontally orientated heart.

The heart has a strong central fibrous skeleton formed largely by four fibrous rings (annulae) that surround the heart valves and separate the atria from the ventricles. The aortic, mitral and tricuspid annulae are intimately related to one another, whilst the pulmonary ring lies higher (Figure 1.2). The skeleton provides a firm anchorage for the attachments of the atrial and ventricular musculature as well as the valvular apparatus. A strong central fibrous body lies between the posterior wall of the aortic root and the upper part of the mitral and tricuspid valves. The inter-atrial septum attaches to the upper part, whilst the lower part becomes continuous with the inter-ventricular septum.

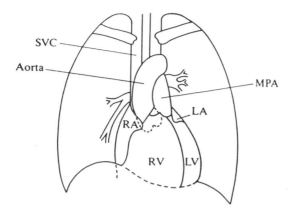

Figure 1.1 Position of heart in the chest. RA = right atrium; LA = left atrium; RV = right ventricle; LV = left ventricle; MPA = main pulmonary artery; SVC = superior vena cava (From Jowett and Thompson: Comprehensive Coronary Care (2nd Ed) 1995. Reproduced by kind permission of Academic Press Ltd London).

The main mass of the heart consists of strong muscular tissue, the myocardium, which is lined on its inner surface by the endocardium and covered externally by the epicardium. The myocardium is composed of a network of specialised involuntary striated myocardial cells which are grouped in bundles in a connective tissue framework. The muscle fibres branch and inter-connect and adjacent cell 'joints' can be seen as thick dark striations called intercalated discs. Because of the close relationship of one muscle fibre with the next, once contraction starts in any part, it cannot remain localised and spreads throughout the entire network of myocardial cells.

There is no muscular continuity between the atria and the ventricles except through the conducting tissue of the atrio-ventricular (AV) node and AV bundle. This specialised conducting tissue comprises modified muscular rather than neural cells.

A tough, fibrous tissue called the pericardium encloses the heart and serves to limit any sudden cardiac distension. On the inner surface of the fibrous pericardium is a thin, delicate membrane called the serous pericardium which extends onto the surface of the heart as the epicardium. The epicardium covers the outer surface of the heart and the adjoining portions of the great vessels. Where the great vessels pass through the pericardium, the two layers of the serous pericardium are reflected back and become continuous with one another. Between the two layers is a potential space, the pericardial cavity, which normally contains a small amount of fluid (20–30 ml) secreted by the serous pericardium which acts as a lubricant to help movement of the heart within the pericardial cavity.

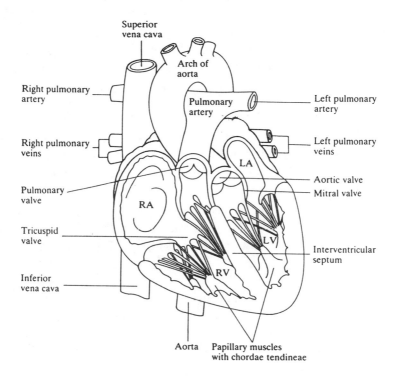

Figure 1.2 The internal anatomy of the heart. RA = right atrium; LA = left atrium; RV = right ventricle; LV = left ventricle (From Jowett and Thompson: Comprehensive Coronary Care (2nd Ed) 1995. Reproduced by kind permission of Academic Press Ltd London).

The pericardium blends with the tunica adventitia of the great vessels and is firmly attached to the central tendon of the diaphragm below and to the back of the sternum by the sterno-pericardial ligaments, thus anchoring the heart within the mediastinum.

The Chambers and Valves of the Heart

The heart consists of four chambers, two atria above and two ventricles below. The junction of the atria and ventricles are marked externally by the atrio-ventricular groove. The right and left sides of the heart are separated by an inter-atrial septum above and an interventricular septum below, and these are marked externally by an anterior and posterior inter-ventricular groove. There are four heart valves, which are designed to allow uni-directional flow of blood through the heart. They are complex avascular structures, and are

very strong. During a normal lifetime they will open and close some
2700 million times. The valves which lie between the atria and ventricles are known as atrio-ventricular (AV) valves. These are the mitral
valve on the left and the tricuspid valve on the right. The semi-lunar
valves are outflow valves from the ventricles and lie at the origins of the
aorta (the aortic valve) and pulmonary artery (the pulmonary valve).

The Atrio-ventricular Valves

The mitral valve lies between the left atrium and left ventricle; the
name derives from the appearance of the two valve leaflets which
resemble a bishop's mitre when they come together. It is the smaller
of the two AV valves, and measures about 9 cm round. The normal
valve orifice is between 4–6 cm². With pathological narrowing of
the valve (mitral stenosis), the valve area is reduced below 2 cm².
Between the right atrium and the right ventricle lies the larger
tricuspid valve, which as its name suggests has three cusps, and
measures about 11 cm in circumference. The AV valves open
passively into the ventricles as blood flows in from the atria during
diastole, and snap shut during systole as pressure in the ventricles
rise. The cusps are prevented from being forced up into the atria
(prolapsing) by strong fibrous cords called chordae tendineae, which
attach to the free edge of the cusps. Tension is applied to these by
special muscles known as papillary muscles which are projections
from the inner wall of the ventricular myocardium and which also
contract in systole. In the condition called 'mitral valve prolapse',
dysfunction of the papillary muscles allows one or both of the mitral
valve leaflets to flop backwards into the left atrium, rendering the
valve incompetent.

The Semi-lunar Valves

The aortic and pulmonary valves are each composed of three 'half-
moon' shaped cusps firmly attached to the fibrous skeleton, and lie at
the exits of the right and left ventricle. They are forced open when
blood is expelled from the heart during ventricular systole. During
diastole, regurgitant flow in the pulmonary artery and aorta causes
the valve cusps to fill like small balloons, forcing the valve edges
tightly together, and preventing flow back into the ventricles.

The aortic valve is about 7.5 cm in circumference and the
pulmonary valve about 1 cm bigger. The aortic valve area is between
2.5–3.5 cm². In the condition known as aortic stenosis, the orifice is
reduced to 1.5 cm² or less.

The pulmonary cusps are referred to as the right anterior, left anterior and posterior cusps according to their position. The three aortic cusps derive their names from their relationship to the coronary arteries, which leave the aorta from the coronary sinuses, which are small pouches situated immediately behind the valve cusps. The names are therefore the right coronary cusp, the left coronary cusp and the non-coronary cusp.

Ventricular Inflow and Outflow Tracts

Blood flows into the ventricles from the atria along special channels called inflow tracts, which extend from the AV valves to the apices of the ventricles. The walls of the tract are trabeculated, more so on the right, and serve to slow blood entering into the ventricles. There are similar modified channels called outflow tracts which extend from the apices of the ventricles to the semi-lunar valves which are smooth walled to help rapid ejection of blood from the heart.

The Cardiac Cycle

The circulation of blood around the body relies on the cyclical pumping action of the heart. Each cycle is normally initiated by spontaneous generation of an impulse (the action potential) at the sino-atrial node. The periods of contraction and relaxation are referred to as systole and diastole. Systole is made up of three phases (iso volumetric contraction, rapid ejection and late systole) and diastole has four phases (iso-volumetric relaxation, rapid filling, passive filling and atrial systole). At a heart rate of 75 beats per minute, the duration of each cardiac cycle is about 0.8 second, with diastole lasting approximately two-thirds of each cycle (0.53 second). As the heart rate increases, both systolic and diastolic timings shorten, but the diastolic period does so proportionally more. For example, at a heart rate of 180 beats/minute, diastole only occupies 40% of the cardiac cycle. The significance of this is that at fast heart rates (particularly abnormal tachycardias), the time available for the diastolic filling of the coronary arteries and ventricles is shortened, which may impair cardiac performance, particularly in patients with cardiac disease.

Atrial filling takes place in diastole, a process which takes about 0.3 second. The AV valves then open, allowing blood to pour into the ventricles which fill up rapidly. The mitral and tricuspid valve cusps float upwards into opposition as the ventricles reach filling capacity, at which point the atria contract, the right atrium a little before the left atrium. Atrial systole takes about 0.1 second, during which an extra 20–40 ml of blood are squeezed into the left ventricle before the mitral valve shuts. The left ventricular end diastolic volume (LVEDV) is approximately 140 ml but will be reduced if the extra contribution from atrial contraction is lost. This situation occurs if there is atrial fibrillation (where the atria do not contract), or when atrial and ventricular contraction are not in sequence (eg. complete heart block). This extra atrial blood may form up to 25% of the LVEDV, thus making a significant contribution the cardiac output. In addition the stretching of the left ventricle when the extra blood is squeezed in has a priming action on the left ventricular wall to ensure a strong ejection beat (the principle of Starling's Law, see below).

Since there are no valves in the venae cavae or at the entrance to the right atrium, some blood is expelled backwards during atrial contraction, causing a transient rise in the central venous pressure – the '*a*' wave of the venous pulse waveform (see Chapter 8).

The AV valves snap shut at the onset of ventricular systole, causing the first heart sound (S1) which may be heard with a stethoscope. The valve cusps are prevented from prolapsing by the pull of the papillary muscles on the chordae tendineae, which ensure that the valve edges are held in close opposition.

During the first phase of ventricular systole, the ventricles contract and change dimensions, becoming shorter and fatter (isovolumetric contraction). This process is the most energy consuming of the whole cardiac cycle, and pressure rises to about 8 mmHg in the right ventricle and 80 mmHg in the left ventricle. The rise in pressure in the right ventricle momentarily causes a backward bulging of the tricuspid valve into the right atrium causing a transient increase in atrial pressure, seen as the '*c*' wave in the venous pulse wave.

The aortic valve opens when the left ventricular pressure exceeds that in the aorta and blood is ejected from the ventricle at first rapidly (rapid ejection phase) and then more slowly (late systole). The AV ring descends to help the ejection of blood and may be seen as the '*x* descent' in the venous pulse wave. At a heart rate of 75 beats/minute, the total systolic period will have lasted about a quarter of a second.

The ventricle does not empty completely, but expels about two-thirds of its contents. This quantity of blood is known as the *stroke volume* and typically ranges from 60–130 ml per beat. The amount of blood left behind is referred to as the end-systolic volume and is about 50 ml. The proportion of LVEDV which has been expelled is called the *ejection fraction*, and is an important index of left ventricular function. In the above example, where the LVEDV was 140 ml, and the stroke volume was 90 ml, the ejection fraction (EF) is thus 90/140 = 64%. Patients with cardiac failure have a reduced ejection fraction, typically less than 40%.

As the ventricles relax, the pressure inside the pulmonary artery and in the aorta falls, and backflow of blood fills the balloon-like semi-lunar valves causing then to close tightly together. Aortic valve closure may be seen as the dicrotic notch on intra-arterial pressure wave recordings (see Chapter 8). The aortic valve normally closes slightly before the pulmonary valve, and this asynchronous valve closure can usually be heard as a split second heart sound (S2) on auscultation. This physiological splitting of the second heart sound can be emphasised by inspiration, when transiently increased blood flow through the right side of the heart slightly delays ventricular emptying and thus pulmonary valve closure.

At the same time as the aortic and pulmonary valves close, blood has once again started to flow into the atria, and intra-atrial pressures start to rise. The AV ring moves back up at the end of ventricular systole producing the '*v* wave' in the venous pulse. When the AV valves open, blood is waiting in the atria to flow rapidly into the ventricles again for the next cycle, sometimes producing an audible third heart sound (S3) in children and young adults as the rapid flow plunges into the left ventricle.

The *cardiac output* is the total volume of blood expelled from the heart in a minute. If the stroke volume is 90 ml, then at a pulse rate of 70 the cardiac output will be 70 x 90 = 6,300 ml = 6.3 litres. The *cardiac index* relates the cardiac output to the patient's size, and it has been found that the best correlation is based upon the body surface area (BSA). The BSA may be determined from a reference chart (Figure 1.3), and the normal cardiac index is then given by:

$$\frac{\text{Cardiac output}}{\text{BSA}} = 2\text{–}5 \text{ litres/minute/metre}^2$$

At rest the cardiac index is about 3.5 l/min/m^2, but may increase rapidly during exertion as heart rate and stroke volume increase.

The right ventricular cardiac cycle is similar to the left ventricular cycle, although timing is different with longer filling and ejection periods. Contraction of the right ventricle occurs later than the left

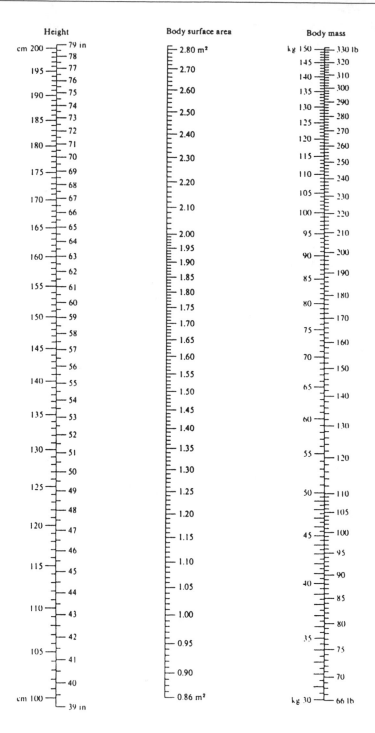

Figure 1.3 Nomogram for estimation of adult body surface area from height and body mass. A straight line should be drawn between the patient's height and weight to reveal the body surface area.

ventricle and is of shorter duration. Right ventricular ejection there-fore begins before and finishes after left ventricular ejection.

The Coronary Circulation (Figure 1.4)

The heart receives its blood supply from right and left coronary arter-ies which originate from two of the three coronary sinuses in the prox-imal aorta. The arteries extend over the epicardial surface of the heart and gives rise to branches which push through the myocardial wall at right-angles to supply the underlying myocardium and endo-cardium. The epicardial supply of blood is therefore more reliable, and less easily compromised than the endocardial supply. In addition, the sub-endocardial portion of the ventricular myocardium is prone to ischaemia because its blood supply in impeded by the high intra-ventricular pressure. This is why minor coronary thrombosis is often associated with sub-endocardial rather than full thickness infarction.

There is much individual variation in the way that the coronary branches supply the various parts of the heart. The left coronary artery generally supplies the majority of the left ventricle and inter-

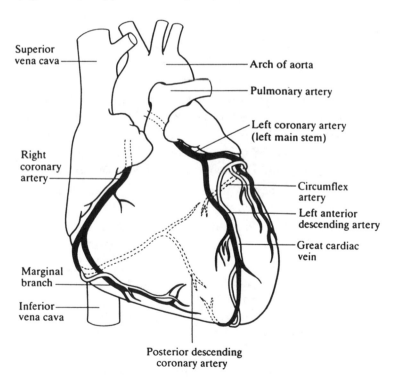

Figure 1.4 The coronary circulation (From Jowett and Thompson: Comprehensive Coronary Care (2nd Ed) 1995. Reproduced by kind permission of Academic Press Ltd London).

ventricular septum including the bundle branches, whilst the right coronary artery supplies most of the right ventricle and the remainder of the conducting tissues.

a) The right coronary artery

The right coronary artery arises from the right coronary sinus, behind the right coronary cusp of the aortic valve. It passes behind the pulmonary artery and runs forward to the atrio-ventricular (AV) groove, encircling the tricuspid valve and usually giving off a small branch to the sino-atrial node. The node is otherwise supplied by a branch of the left coronary artery. The right coronary artery then passes downwards and around the inferior border of the heart, giving off a prominent acute marginal branch to supply the wall of the right ventricle. It then winds round to the back of the heart and passes down in the inter-ventricular groove as the posterior descending coronary artery which supplies the posterior aspect of both ventricles, the atrio-ventricular node, and the inter-ventricular septum. Frequently, a transverse branch continues straight on in the posterior AV groove, supplying the left atrium before anastomosing with the circumflex branch of the left coronary artery.

b) The left coronary artery

The left coronary artery arises from the left coronary sinus behind the left coronary cusp of the aortic valve, and runs forwards as the left main stem coronary artery between the pulmonary artery and the left atrial appendage to the AV groove. Here, it divides into two branches – the left anterior descending branch and the left circumflex branch. These two arteries with the right coronary artery make up the three arteries referred to in 'triple artery disease'.

The left anterior descending artery (LAD) descends in the anterior inter-ventricular groove to the apex of the heart, where it turns under to ascend a short distance up the posterior inter-ventricular groove, anastomosing with the posterior inter-ventricular branch of the right coronary artery. Diagonal branches supply the anterior ventricular wall, and septal branches supply the inter-ventricular septum and the bundle branches.

The left circumflex branch is very variable. It passes round the left margin of the heart in the AV groove under the left atrial appendage, giving off branches to the left atrium and occasionally the branch to the sino-atrial node. Obtuse marginal branches supply the lateral aspect of the heart, one of which may arise directly from the left coronary artery to form a trifurcation rather than a bifurcation at the termination of the left main stem. This vessel is then called the first obtuse marginal artery. Postero-lateral branches of the circumflex artery supply the posterior and inferior walls of the left ventricle. Sometimes the circumflex artery continues right around the left border of the heart to give rise to the posterior descending and AV nodal arteries. The left coronary artery will then supply the inferior surface of the heart, along with the entire supply to the inter-ventricular septum. This is called a left dominant system.

When applied to the coronary circulation 'vessel dominance' does not imply the larger of the two coronary arteries, but is applied to whichever artery crosses the intersection of the inter-atrial and inter-ventricular grooves and the AV groove at the back of the heart to supply the inferior surface of the heart and septum. Thus, in 85% of individuals, it is the right coronary artery which is dominant, although it is the left coronary artery which is usually of wider calibre, supplying the larger part of the myocardium.

Coronary Blood Flow

The primary function of the coronary circulation is to provide an adequate supply of oxygen to support the metabolic needs of the heart. Approximately 5% of the cardiac output passes into the coronary vessels (about 275 ml/minute) which fill in diastole. During systole, the coronary vessels are compressed, so that resistance to flow increases sharply. The rate of oxygen consumption is a major factor in determining blood flow, which in turn is determined by such variables as heart rate, intra-myocardial tension and the degree of myofibril shortening. Low oxygen levels are a very potent coronary vasodilator. Myocardial oxygen consumption normally increases during exercise, and may additionally rise in response to other stimuli, including drugs such as adrenaline, calcium, thyroxine and digoxin. A reduction in the size of the arterial lumen by atheromatous deposits or spasm can markedly inhibit flow. For example, a reduction in diameter by as little as 25% can increase resistance to flow by a factor of eight.

A *coronary collateral circulation* is present within the heart. This is produced by inter-arterial vessels which connect two branches of a single coronary artery, or connect branches of the right coronary artery to branches of the left coronary artery. They are present from birth, but are not functionally significant until there is coronary ischaemia or ventricular hypertrophy. From poorly developed, narrow vessels, these collateral vessels can change into fully functioning arterioles with significant enlargement being seen within as little as nine days following an ischaemic event. These collateral vessels may regress following successful coronary re-vascularisation by angioplasty or bypass surgery.

Patients with long-standing stable angina often have a well developed collateral circulation, so that acute coronary thrombosis is often associated with a smaller myocardial infarction than would have occurred in those patients with no previous symptoms, and who thus possess an under-developed collateral circulation.

The coronary veins run with the coronary arteries. Those draining blood from the distribution of the left coronary artery terminate in the coronary sinus which lies in the diaphragmatic part of the AV groove. This then empties into the right atrium. Blood from the territory of the right coronary artery drains mainly into the anterior cardiac veins, which also drain into the right atrium. Coronary venous blood is almost completely de-saturated since virtually all the oxygen is extracted by coronary capillaries.

The Nerve Supply to the Heart

Heart transplantation operations have shown that the heart has the ability to function without innervation. Its 'intrinsic rhythmicity' allows it to beat without external control, even when completely removed from the body. However, the heart is well supplied with both sympathetic and parasympathetic nerve fibres which can modify cardiac function by changing the rate and strength of myocardial contraction.

The sympathetic fibres derive from the cervical and upper thoracic sympathetic ganglia and the parasympathetic supply from the vagus nerves. The vagal and sympathetic nerves are distributed to the heart by the cardiac plexus which lies between the concavity of the aortic arch and the tracheal bifurcation.

Sympathetic nerve fibres supply both the conducting tissues and the myocardial cells. Sympathetic stimulation accelerates the discharge rate of the sino-atrial (SA) node, enhances conduction through the atrio-ventricular (AV) node and increases the force of myocardial contraction. Release of catecholamines (adrenaline/noradrenaline) from the adrenal medulla may also produce the same effect on the heart.

Parasympathetic nerve fibres supply mainly the SA node and AV node and to a lesser extent the atrial and ventricular musculature. Stimulation of these parasympathetic nerves slows the heart rate, reduces the force of myocardial contraction, and slows conduction through the AV node.

Sensory impulses travel from the myocardium via sympathetic fibres to the thoracic sympathetic ganglia of spinal nerve roots T1–T5. The sensory distribution of these nerves is to the anterior chest wall and the inner aspect of the arm and hand. Cardiac pain is therefore usually felt in the territory of these thoracic nerves, and rarely extends beyond the region bounded by the lower jaw and the epigastrium (C3–T6 dermatomes).

Cardiac performance can also be affected by special sensory receptors called baro-receptors which detect pressure changes in the aorta and carotid arteries. Excessive pressure in these vessels causes stimulation of the baro-receptors which then feed back to slow the heart, reduce the cardiac output and thus lower the blood pressure. This aortic reflex helps maintain a normal arterial blood pressure.

Artificial stimulation of the baro-receptors by carotid sinus massage is used clinically to slow the heart during supra-ventricular tachycardias.

Similar receptors are found in the venae cavae which are stimulated by increased venous return. This produces sympathetic stimulation of the heart to increase the heart rate. In contrast, reduced venous flow in the venae cavae is associated with parasympathetic stimulation which slows the heart rate. This auto-regulation of the heart rate to deal with variations in venous return is known as the 'Bainbridge reflex'.

The Conducting System

In addition to the purely contractile muscle fibres, the heart possesses certain specialised muscle cells which form the conducting system. These are 'automatic cells' which are able to initiate and conduct electrical impulses within the heart to produce myocardial contraction. The conducting system (Figure 1.5) comprises:

1)   The sino-atrial (SA) node
2)   The atrio-ventricular (AV) junction
        The AV node
        The Bundle of His
3)   The bundle branches
        Right and left bundle branches
        Purkinje fibres.

The normal sequence of conduction is initiated by an electrical impulse arising at the sino-atrial node. The impulse is transmitted

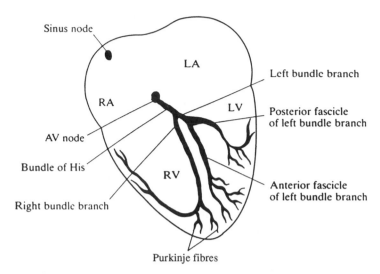

Sinus node

LA

Left bundle branch

RA

LV

Posterior fascicle
of left bundle branch

AV node

Bundle of His

RV

Right bundle branch

Anterior fascicle
of left bundle branch

Purkinje fibres

Figure 1.5 The conducting tissues of the heart (From Jowett and Thompson: Comprehensive Coronary Care (2nd Ed) 1995. Reproduced by kind permission of Academic Press Ltd London).

via specialised atrial conducting pathways to the atrio-ventricular node, depolarizing the atria as it passes through. There is a slight delay in transmission here which allows atrial systole to complete before the ventricles are depolarized. The impulse rapidly travels down the bundle branches to the Purkinje fibres and into the ventricular myocardium. The septum is the first part of the ventricular mass to be depolarized, and is so from left to right. The remainder of the myocardium is then depolarized, with the depolarizing wave spreading outwards from the endocardium to the epicardium.

1) The sino-atrial node

The sino-atrial node is the normal site for initiation of the heart beat. It is a small cigar-shaped structure located between the openings of the superior and inferior vena cavae within the wall of the right atrium. There are numerous autonomic nerve endings in the node including parasympathetic fibres derived from the right vagus nerve. The blood supply is from the nodal artery, which in most people arises from the right coronary artery.

2) The atrio-ventricular junction

The atrio-ventricular (AV) junction comprises the AV node and the Bundle of His. The AV node lies in the right atrial wall between the opening of the coronary sinus and the posterior border of the membranous inter-ventricular septum. It causes a delay in transmission of the cardiac impulse from the atria to the ventricles so that the atria have had time to expel their contents into the ventricles before they contract.

There is a rich autonomic nerve supply to the AV node with parasympathetic fibres derived from the left vagus nerve. The major blood supply to the atrial component of the AV junction is from a nodal artery which arises from the right posterior descending coronary artery in 90% of people, and from the left circumflex artery in the remaining 10%. The supply to the ventricular conduction segments comes from the septal perforating branches of the left anterior descending coronary artery. The bundle of His extends from the AV node, along the posterior margin of the membranous portion of the inter-ventricular septum and bifurcates into the right and left bundle branches on reaching the muscular part of the septum.

3) The bundle branches

The right and left bundle branches extend sub-endocardially along both sides of the inter-ventricular septum. The right bundle is a cord-like structure which passes down the right side of the inter-ventricular septum towards the apex, lying more deeply beneath the endocardium than does the left main bundle. It ramifies amongst the right ventricular musculature near the base of the anterior papillary muscle.

The left bundle branch is a sheet of fibres which pass down the left side of the inter-ventricular septum. The initial part of the left bundle is fan shaped, which breaks up into left and right hemi-fascicles. The terminal branches of the bundle branches are the Purkinje fibres which ramify sub-endocardially within the ventricular mass.

Cardiac Performance

The ability of the heart to maintain an adequate cardiac output is dependent on an adequate cardiac performance. Cardiac performance is determined by four main factors:

a)   Pre-load (filling of the heart in diastole)
b)   Afterload (resistance against which blood must be ejected)
c)   Contractility of the heart muscle
d)   Heart rate.

a) Pre-load

Pre-load is the degree of tension exerted on cardiac muscle immediately prior to the onset of systole, and is usually expressed as the left ventricular end-diastolic pressure (LVEDP). This is in turn determined by the volume of blood in the ventricle at that time, the left ventricular end-diastolic volume (LVEDV) which is influenced by venous return. Because the volume of blood being returned to the heart may vary considerably, the cardiac muscle can vary the force of contraction to maintain the ejection fraction. According to Starling's Law, the more that the myocardial cells are stretched, the more forcefully they will contract (within physiological limits). Hence, the larger the LVEDV, the more stretch will be applied to the heart, the stronger the force of subsequent contraction, and the bigger the stroke volume. This intrinsic ability of the heart to adapt to changing load may be shown graphically (Figure 1.6), and is approximately linear. However, once the load increases beyond physiological limits, the heart fails, and the heart is unable to increase the degree of contraction regardless of fibre stretch.

The optimal pre-load for the left ventricle is between 6-12 mmHg. However, this figure may vary when influenced by factors or pathological processes which affect ventricular compliance (stiffness). For example, following acute myocardial infarction patients may develop stiffening of the left ventricular wall, and a higher pre-load may be required to overcome the resistance to ventricular distensibility. The reverse is seen in dilated cardiomyopathies, where abnormal compliance of the flabby ventricles reduce the pre-load requirements for optimal cardiac performance.

Atrial stretch receptors may also help by signalling to the adrenal medulla which then releases catecholamines to additionally stimulate the heart rate and force of contraction.

Clinically, pre-load may be estimated by measuring the atrial

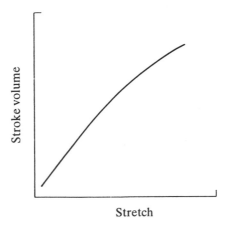

Figure 1.6 Starling's Law graph (From Jowett and Thompson: Comprehensive Coronary Care (2nd Ed) 1995. Reproduced by kind permission of Academic Press Ltd London)

pressures, either by the a central venous pressure (CVP) line to measure the right atrial pressure, or a Swan-Ganz catheter to measure the left atrial pressure.

b) Afterload

Afterload refers to the force opposing the ejection of blood from the ventricles. The most critical factor determining afterload is vascular resistance, although any pathological resistance from the semi-lunar valves needs taking into account (eg. aortic stenosis). Afterload therefore usually equates with the systemic vascular resistance (SVR) and pulmonary vascular resistance (PVR). A high afterload makes the ejection of blood more difficult, and increases the amount of myocardial work needed to overcome the resistance. As a result, as afterload changes, reciprocal changes are seen in the stroke volume and myocardial oxygen consumption.

'Off-loading' the heart is a term used in the management of cardiac failure where drug treatment is used to vasodilate arteries, reducing the ejection force required to empty the left ventricle thus raising the stroke volume and improving the cardiac output.

c) Myocardial contractility

Contractility (inotropism) is an intrinsic property of the heart, and exists whether or not it is stretched by filling with blood. The speed and force of contraction (positive chronotropism and inotropism) can be increased by sympathetic nerve stimulation, or by drugs such as adrenaline and dopamine. The Frank-Starling curve is displaced upwards and to the right (Figure 1.7). Myocardial hypoxia and beta-

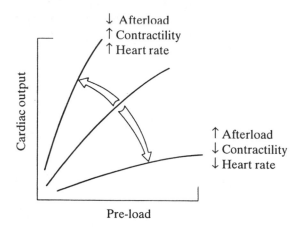

Figure 1.7 Frank Starling curves showing the effects of preload, afterload, contractility and heart rate (From Jowett and Thompson: Comprehensive Coronary Care (2nd Ed) 1995. Reproduced by kind permission of Academic Press Ltd London)

blocking agents have the opposite effect, and decrease both heart rate (negatively chronotropic) and force of contraction (negatively inotropic).

Contractility also needs to be coordinated for optimal cardiac performance. The extreme example of incoordination is during ventricular fibrillation when there is no cardiac output. Other reasons may include myocardial ischaemia or myocardial infarction where injured or dead muscle will not contract properly.

The strength of contraction may be gauged by the size of the ejection fraction which can be determined by echocardiography, nuclear scanning or at cardiac catheterisation. These techniques will additionally give information about the coordination and efficiency of ventricular contraction.

d) Heart rate

The heart rate is largely dependent upon the balance of sympathetic and parasympathetic activity, and is normally directly related to the metabolic rate. The healthy heart rate can vary its speed within seconds to help vary the cardiac output, but very fast heart rates may be associated with a reduction in cardiac performance, since ventricular filling time and coronary perfusion are decreased. Abnormal rhythms such as atrial fibrillation and complete heart block reduce ventricular filling because of the loss of atrial systole, or because of asynchrony of AV contraction, and are also associated with a reduced cardiac output.

Chapter 2
Cardiovascular Monitoring: Clinical or Technical?

Utilising complex equipment for cardiovascular monitoring is no substitute for the bedside appraisal of the patient. Making therapeutic decisions based solely on data from machines, rather than on clinical judgement, is extremely dangerous. It is important to consider the clinical history and the physical findings, although full evaluation will often be influenced by information obtainable by monitoring techniques. If invasive studies are needed, safe patient management demands that only appropriate monitoring is carried out, thus avoiding unnecessary increases in the hazards of cardiovascular monitoring and the costs of such interventions.

A: Clinical observations

There are a number of general observations that can be made at the bedside which may help in the overall assessment of the patient. Evaluating the level of distress or discomfort is an obvious initial step; further observations will be made difficult if not impossible unless pain is relieved. Other general observations might include the state of nutrition and hydration, skin colour and temperature, distension of the neck veins, shortness of breath, level of consciousness and appropriateness of speech.

Level of Consciousness

The level of consciousness and mental status is a valuable guide to the overall condition of the patient, and changes may be of critical importance. Agitation, distress, state of alertness and communicativeness are valuable adjuncts to more objective physiological data.

The *Glasgow Coma Scale* (GCS) is a widely used method for monitoring changing levels of consciousness. Each time the patient is examined, a score is estimated which will fall within the range of 3 (the worst) to 15 (the best). This score is made up from three groups of responses (Table 2.1).

Whilst this scale has been primarily developed to evaluate patients with cerebral trauma, it may be used for rapid evaluation of acutely or severely ill patients, particularly if their status is changing frequently.

It must be noted the any assessment of coma will be adversely influenced by certain drugs, such as neuro-muscular blocking agents, or those which depress the central nervous system.

Shortness of Breath

Bedside assessment of ventilation may be made by observing the patient's colour, respiratory rate and adequacy of chest movement. The respiratory rate should be counted over at least 30 seconds, and the depth of respiration noted. Obvious dyspnoea may be caused by such factors as pain, anxiety, cardiac failure, respiratory tract infection, hypoxaemia or acidaemia.

Table 2.1: The Glasgow Coma Scale

I)   Best eye opening response
     Spontaneous = 4
     To speech = 3
     To pain = 2
     No response = 1

II) Best motor response
     Obeys commands = 6
     Localises stimuli = 5
     Withdraws from stimulus = 4
     Abnormal flexion (decorticate) response = 3
     Abnormal extension (decerebrate) response = 2
     No response = 1

III) Best verbal response
     Oriented = 5
     Confused conversation = 4
     Inappropriate words = 3
     Incomprehensible sounds = 2
     No response = 1

     Best response = 15   Worst response = 3

The Skin

Repeated assessment of skin colour, temperature, moisture and turgor are useful bedside observations. Skin temperature provides a valuable indication of cutaneous blood flow, and measurement of skin temperature is widely used in high dependency units for monitoring changes in cardiac output in response to treatment. In low output states, such as cardiac failure or hypo-volaemic shock, the skin will be cool and clammy, whilst in high cardiac output states (eg. septicaemic shock or thyrotoxicosis) the skin is usually warm.

Capillary refill time can also provide an assessment of peripheral blood flow. Normally, the nail bed blanches when the fingernail is pressed, which then becomes pink almost immediately on release of pressure indicating good peripheral perfusion. In patients with poor peripheral perfusion, this pinking process takes much longer.

Pallor may indicate anaemia, or may be seen in low output states when blood is diverted away from the skin as a result of sympathetically mediated vaso-constriction.

Cyanosis describes the blue (cyan) discolouration of the skin and mucous membranes caused by excessive concentrations of reduced (deoxygenated) oxygen. Cyanosis may be described as either peripheral or central.

Peripheral cyanosis occurs at the peripheries of the body (the fingers and toes) and is caused by a higher degree of oxygen extraction at those sites. It usually indicates a slowing of peripheral circulation, allowing more oxygen to be extracted as the blood passes through the constricted capillaries and occurs most commonly when the patient is cold. In hospital practice it is often seen in patients with low output states such as shock or cardiac failure when there is sympathetically mediated cutaneous vaso-constriction.

Central cyanosis is observed centrally in the body, ie. in the lips and tongue. It is caused by inadequate oxygenation of the blood as it passes through the lungs, as in pulmonary disease and pulmonary oedema or sometimes when the lungs are bypassed all together (as with ventriculo-septal defects). These latter patients usually have clubbing of the fingers and toes.

Rarely, central cyanosis can be produced by certain drugs which cause the formation of methaemoglobin and sulphaemoglobin.

Absence of cyanosis does not exclude hypoxaemia; when in doubt, oxygen or assisted ventilation should be given.

Skin turgor may be an important guide to hydration. A dry tongue may indicate dehydration or mouth breathing. Picking up a fold of skin beneath the clavicle is a better guide. Normal skin folds drop back immediately, whereas the skin of dehydrated patients remains puckered. Using skin on the back of the hand for this test is not advised. In elderly patients skin elasticity is lost and a false positive response may be obtained.

Oedema

Oedema is the presence of fluid in the tissues. Oedema which pits in response to pressure by the fingers is an important sign of salt and fluid overload, especially in cardiac failure. The fluid accumulates in the most dependent body position, so for patients in bed, this is usually over the sacrum, although in ambulant patients it will be the ankles. As fluid overload worsens, the legs and genitalia may become swollen, and later there will be ascites and pleural effusions.

Other causes of oedema include hypo-albuminaemia, venous stasis and conditions associated with elevated right heart pressures.

B: Cardiovascular Monitoring – Clinical

Whilst general observations can reveal a great deal about the patient's current status, simple clinical monitoring techniques can greatly enhance the evaluation of the patient, without resorting to expensive electronic equipment.

Vital signs

The body temperature, pulse and respiratory rate (TPR), along with blood pressure, are termed the vital signs, and are the most commonly measured physiological variables in clinical practice. They form very useful baseline observations in all patients, and are the usual parameters measured during daily nursing routines. Such signs should be recorded more frequently in the acute period of an illness to provide a graphic record for evaluation of the patient's changing condition.

a) Temperature

Body temperature is a non-specific variable. The normal oral temperature is considered to be 37°C (98.4°F), but many normal individuals demonstrate a diurnal variation in temperature, perhaps varying between 36–37.5°C. Whilst recording and monitoring the body temperature is extremely useful in many patients, it is particularly valuable in patients recovering from hypothermia (eg. following cardiac surgery).

The body temperature is usually taken with a mercury thermometer placed in the axilla or under the tongue. The latter is preferable unless the patient is unconscious or unable to close his mouth. A new development has been the introduction and widespread use of electronic thermometers. Oral electronic thermometers utilise a disposable probe which is placed under the tongue and when removed and connected to a special handle will produce an accurate temperature reading within a minute (Graftemp, Astra). A much faster estimation may be made by an aural electronic thermometer which uses a probe placed gently in the external auditory meatus until a seal is made (Genius, Sherwood Medical). Infra-red temperature measurements are made from the tympanic membrane which, because it shares a blood supply with the hypothalamus in the brain (the temperature control centre), provides an accurate body core temperature within seconds.

For patients in the intensive care unit, a skin sensor and/or an electronic probe inserted into the rectum is often of greater value, since it can provide a continuous read-out of body temperature. Rectal temperatures are considered core temperatures, and are on average 0.6°C higher than oral temperatures. The core–peripheral temperature gradient is one useful index of adequacy of peripheral perfusion. This is the recorded temperature difference between the rectal probe and the cutaneous probe. It increases when there is vaso-constriction in response to a low cardiac output, and decreases with vaso-dilatation and with an increased cardiac output.

Pyrexia is usually associated with infection, but high temperatures may also be found where there is tissue necrosis, neoplastic disease or hyper-metabolic states.

b) The arterial pulse

The arterial pulse is generated by left ventricular systolic contraction. A great deal of information can be gathered from palpation of the pulse, including rate, rhythm, character and symmetry.

Pulse rate

The pulse rate is usually taken by palpation of the radial pulse and the rate estimated over 30 seconds, or longer if the pulse is irregular. In patients with atrial fibrillation, it is better to assess the pulse rate by listening to the patient's heart which gives the ventricular rate, since weaker beats will not be transmitted to the peripheries. Taking the apex–radial pulse rate (comparison of the apical and radial pulse rates) is useful in assessing rate control in atrial fibrillation.

In patients on bedside monitors, the ventricular heart rate is usually displayed automatically, being calculated from either the ECG tracing or arterial waveform.

The normal adult pulse rate varies between 60–100 beats per minute, and is a non-specific cardio-respiratory variable. Slower rates (bradycardias) are often found in athletes, and are found in patients taking certain cardiac drugs, such as beta-adrenergic blocking agents, diltiazem or verapamil. Fast pulse rates (tachycardias) may be associated with anxiety, fever, exercise and pain as well as giving some indication of a compromised circulatory status. Resting pulse rates above 130/minute usually indicate an abnormal tachycardia.

Apart from the rate, arterial pulses can be examined for rhythm, volume and character of the waveform. Although the rate and rhythm are usually assessed by palpation of the radial artery, an artery closer to the heart is usually better for appreciating pulse volume and character of the waveform. In clinical practice, all features may be best assessed by palpation of the right brachial artery.

Pulse rhythm

The normal pulse is regular, or very slightly irregular if there is a sinus arrythmia when the heart quickens on inspiration. An occasional irregularity indicates an ectopic beat, and an irregularly irregular pulse either indicates multifocal ectopic beats or atrial fibrillation. Gently exercising the patient will produce a regular pulse in the former cases (the resulting rise in the pulse rate will abolish the ectopic) whilst it will have no effect on the irregularity produced by atrial fibrillation.

Pulse volume

Pulse volume (width or amplitude) is an appreciation of the pulse pressure (ie. the difference between systolic and diastolic blood pressures). This is described as normal, small or large. Small volume pulses are typically felt in shocked patient, whereas large volume pulses are found in patients with anaemia, thyrotoxicosis or in those who are pregnant.

Character of the pulse waveform

This is not often easily appreciated, but can help with diagnosis. Examples of such descriptions include:

- Pulsus alternans: alternate high and low volume beats as found in left ventricular failure. It indicates poor left ventricular function.

- Pulsus paradoxus: an excessive reduction in pulse pressure (> 10 mmHg) on inspiration. It may be found in asthma, pericardial tamponade or pericardial constriction.
- Collapsing pulse: large volume with rapid rise and fall as may occur in thyrotoxicosis or aortic incompetence.
- Plateau pulse: low volume, slow rise and slow fall, as found in aortic stenosis.
- Absent pulse: due to atherosclerosis, aortic dissection or peripheral embolisation. It is advisable to check for pulse symmetry.

c) Respiratory rate

The rate and pattern of respiration should be observed for 30–60 seconds. The normal respiratory rate at rest is between 10–14 per minute. Many patients hyperventilate when being watched, although a respiratory rate of over 20/minute is probably abnormal. Deep sighs during normal respiration are not uncommon, but an irregular pattern of breathing with multiple sighs usually reflect psychogenic breathlessness, which may sometimes be accompanied by associated complaints induced by the hyperventilation, such as dizziness, parasthaesiae and chest pain.

Orthopnoea is shortness of breath on lying down, and is an important symptom of heart failure. Kussmaul breathing describes rapid, deep respiration, and is an important sign of acidaemia. Cheyne-Stokes breathing is a regular alternating cycle of rapid and slow respiration over 30 seconds or more, often ending with an apnoeic phase. It may associate with cardio-respiratory disorders, or central lesions particularly those affecting the brain stem.

Arterial Blood Pressure

The assessment of the arterial blood pressure is discussed in detail in Chapter 8. As part of a baseline examination, the arterial blood pressure is normally assessed using a mercury or aneroid sphygmomanometer, but electronically operated machines are being utilised more frequently now, with invasive monitoring usually reserved for high dependency areas.

Whilst the blood pressure is diagnostically non-specific, it does provide an index of the overall circulatory status. Low or falling blood pressures indicate circulatory decompensation or failure of a specific therapy, whilst a rising blood pressure usually implies improved circulatory function. The blood pressure does not directly measure changes in blood flow or volume, but simply the adequacy of circulatory compensation. Hence, blood pressure measurements are very useful for screening, and for rapid assessment of trends in emergency conditions, especially trauma, internal bleeding or following acute myocardial infarction.

The normal blood pressure in the healthy adult is about 120/80 mmHg, and gradually increases with age. However, knowledge of the normal blood pressure for the individual is probably more important during haemodynamic monitoring. Many normal young adults may have blood pressures of 90/60 mmHg, and clearly this cannot be diagnosed as shock, although it would be viewed far more seriously in a patient following myocardial infarction or gastro-intestinal haemorrhage.

The *pulse pressure* is the difference between the systolic and diastolic blood pressure, and is often more informative. A fall in pulse pressure often precedes a fall in the diastolic pressure in patients developing hypo-volaemic shock, and is thus an early sign of blood volume loss. Similarly, the return to a normal pulse pressure is often an early sign of successful restoration of circulatory volume.

The *mean arterial pressure* (MAP) is not the sum of the systolic plus the diastolic pressure divided by two, but is an indication of the average perfusion pressure created by the blood pressure over the complete cardiac cycle. It can be calculated directly during intra-arterial monitoring, but may be otherwise estimated by adding the diastolic pressure to one-third of the pulse pressure. The MAP is used to calculate other parameters such as cardiac work and systemic vascular (peripheral) resistance.

Jugular Venous Pressure (JVP)

The level of blood in the internal jugular vein is a guide to the central venous pressure (CVP). Much has been written about the pulsation in the jugular vein, but clinically it is difficult to appreciate, and it is seldom of assistance. Sometimes '*a*' and '*v*' waves may be seen which correspond to atrial and ventricular contraction, and these are much more apparent on a CVP pressure trace.

The internal jugular vein may be seen in front of the sterno-mastoid muscle, although with a normal CVP, pulsation in the vein is usually only visible when the patient lies nearly flat. When observing for elevation, the height above the sternal angle should be measured with the patient lying at 45 degrees, when the maximal level of normality is 4 cm (equivalent to a right atrial pressure of 6 mmHg). Confirmation of the level may be made by pressing on the abdomen which increases the CVP transiently (by increasing venous return to the heart), and produces 'hepato-jugular reflux'. If the JVP is not visible, especially after pressing on the abdomen in the recumbent patient, hypo-volaemia is likely.

The most important abnormality of the JVP is elevation which is an indication of high right-sided cardiac pressures (eg. congestive cardiac failure, cor pulmonale, pulmonary embolism).

Urinary Output

In the absence of intrinsic renal disease, the hourly urine output is a good guide to the adequacy of tissue perfusion. A satisfactory production of urine implies that perfusion of other vital organs is likely to be sufficient. In patients requiring critical care, it is usual to measured hourly volumes via an indwelling catheter and a urimeter. A urine production rate of 0.5–1 ml/kg/hour is deemed satisfactory.

Invasive haemodynamic monitoring can often be withheld if the urinary output is good, especially if the mental state is preserved. If the urinary output falls significantly following haemodynamic stabilisation, it is likely to indicate the onset of acute renal failure.

C: Cardiovascular Monitoring – Technical

Whilst bedside observation of the patient with clinical judgement will always remain of paramount importance, the physiological status of critically ill patients may often change in subtle ways which may not be easily defined clinically, and advanced cardiovascular monitoring may overcome many of these difficulties. Many studies have found that even experienced clinicians may be unable to recognise effective ventilation or detect hypoxaemia adequately. The development of electronic equipment for patient monitoring has overcome many of these difficulties, and is now an integral and essential part of routine and critical care.

The major purpose of monitoring is to recognise and evaluate potential physiological problems as soon as possible, so that therapy may be modified. Cardiovascular monitoring devices have been designed for rapid, frequent, repetitive measurements of physiological variables. Technical developments in recent years have lead to a vast array of monitoring systems, many of which are now in routine use on most high dependency units. Some monitoring techniques are also used for diagnostic purposes (eg. pulmonary artery catheterisation), so that the differentiation between monitoring and diagnosis may be indistinct.

Whatever system is utilised, a thorough knowledge of the systems capabilities and drawbacks is vital. Artifacts are universal and may arise in any part of the system. Sensors are usually subject to patient movement or tremor. Fluid filled catheter systems may be subject to kinking or blocking and electrical interference may distort the signal or read-out.

Electrical safety must be paramount for the sake of both the patient and the staff. The combination of multiple fluid lines and cables in a small area is potentially dangerous, and all must be aware of possible hazards and the safety procedures which may be adopted to avoid the associated risk.

Types of Cardiovascular Monitoring Equipment

All monitoring systems comprise the same key elements:

1   A sensor to detect the signal
2   A transducer to convert the signal into an electrical form
3   A monitor which displays and records the signal.

Whilst it may be necessary to monitor different variables in different patients, the following modalities are usual:

Cardiovascular System:
      Electrocardiogram (ECG)
      Arterial blood pressure
      Central venous pressure (CVP)
      Left atrial pressure (PA wedge pressure)
      Pulmonary artery pressures
      Cardiac output
Respiratory System:
      Respiratory rate
      Oxygen saturation
      Blood gases
Renal system:
      Urinary output
      Blood pH and acid–base status

Most patients can easily be monitored by routine assessment of the vital signs, with an ECG monitor and pulse oximeter if needed. Insertion of CVP lines is commonplace on medical and surgical wards, but other forms of invasive monitoring should perhaps be reserved for high dependency areas.

A simple compact vital signs monitor (Figure 2.1) will allow simultaneous recording of the ECG, blood pressure (non-invasively), oxygen saturation and body temperature, and may be connected to the patient in minutes. When many different parameters are being assessed, these may all be processed by a larger multi-channel monitor, with recordings displayed either individually or in groups.

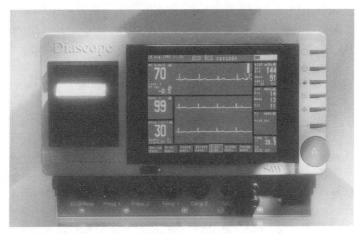

Figure 2.1 Small bedside monitor (Reproduced by kind permission of Vickers Medical, Sidcup, Kent

Machines which record on eight different channels that give 12 different displays are now commonplace. For example, a monitor displaying a cardiovascular profile may exhibit the ECG, the CVP, the systemic and pulmonary arterial pressures as well as the oxygen saturation on the same screen (Figure 2.2).

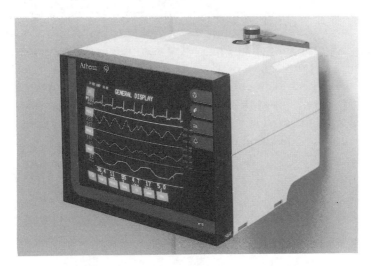

Figure 2.2 Larger multi-channel monitor (Reproduced by kind permission of Vickers Medical, Sidcup, Kent

The Role of the Computer

Intensive care nursing staff spend 20% of their time charting observations derived from monitors, and both they and their doctor colleagues must spend further time in trying to comprehend the vast amount of information. Computer systems are now commonly utilised to analyse, store and record the large amount of physiological data provided by the various monitoring devices. Haemodynamic monitoring is particularly suitable for on-line monitoring, with the ECG, blood pressure, central venous pressure and pulmonary artery pressure all displayed and simultaneously recorded on computer. Trend analysis of measured parameters is now easily achieved whereby a time scale compressed record can be viewed easily, and allows access to retrospective data collected over the preceding 24 hours. With networking techniques, it is possible to have one central monitoring base connected to a hundred or more different beds around the hospital.

Many pathology laboratories are now linked by computer to the wards and high dependency units to save time in transmitting results, thus eliminating errors in recording verbal messages. In addition, it is possible to call up not only the latest result, but also previous results too.

'Expert systems' are evolving whereby artificial intelligence can advise on specific data collected by the system. Further development will help make available the relevant information to those who need it, and in an easily understood format.

As yet, the development and use of computers for patient monitoring has been slow. Some of these problems have been organisational and some financial. The cost of computer hardware has fallen dramatically, but the cost of specialised software remains high. Much of the delay in implementation of computer systems surrounds the required changes in work practice, and acceptance of the role which technology can provide. Computer literacy is generally improving, but continuing education is essential.

Chapter 3
Electrocardio-
graphic Monitoring

Electrocardiographic monitoring is the most common form of continuous cardiovascular monitoring used in hospitals. The original bulky oscilloscopes have been replaced by small refined electronic monitors, with different levels of capabilities.

There are two basic modes of continuous ECG monitoring. The most common is hard wire monitoring which requires the patient to be physically linked via a cable to the bedside monitor. The alternative is telemetry where the patient carries a battery powered transmitter, to relay the ECG signal to a receiver which may be remote. This is useful for continuous ECG monitoring of ambulatory patients.

The bedside monitor will have either a single or multi-lead display. Those with single lead displays often have a second trace underneath which cascades down from the upper trace, thus forming a delayed recording which can be captured for further analysis. Multi-lead displays can demonstrate three different ECG leads simultaneously, but require up to five chest electrodes. Such arrangements may be very useful in the clarification of complex dysrhythmias.

On intensive care and coronary care units, the ECG monitor is usually part of a fixed multi-parameter display, which includes other information being collated, such as intra-cardiac pressures and oxygen saturation. Each bed is linked to a central station where all the data is duplicated on one main screen. This usually houses the heart of the cardiac monitoring system, comprising the computer, hard copy recorder (for recording rhythm strips) and alarm systems. On medical wards, less sophisticated equipment is used and central monitoring is usually not undertaken. A portable monitor is then placed beside the bed of each patient as required. This may be for ECG monitoring alone, although other simple parameters can also be recorded (eg. pulse oximetry, non-invasive blood pressure recording) if an appropriate monitor is utilised.

As may be anticipated, the benefits of electrocardiographic monitoring depend upon whether all potentially serious dysrhythmias are seen and recognised. Although visual observation of the monitor by trained staff is usual, many dysrhythmias are missed because of fatigue, boredom or distraction. The use of computers for detecting and storing dysrhythmias is now commonplace in acute care areas, and certainly highly desirable in other places. These computer-linked monitors are able to recognise many dysrhythmias and sound alarms appropriately. Automatic ECG analysis can be performed at various levels of sophistication from simple ectopic counts to specific dysrhythmia recognition. Graded alarm systems ensure that life-threatening situations take priority over warning or advisory conditions (detached leads, loose cuffs, etc). Using a storage mode, episodes of rhythm disturbance can be recalled, as well as histograms giving trend analysis for each 24 hour period.

There are several considerations for maximising the value of electrocardiographic monitoring. These include:

a)   Knowledge of chest electrode placement and care
b)   Knowing how to set up and operate the monitor
c)   Recognising and distinguishing normal and abnormal rhythms.

How the ECG Waveform is Generated

The normal cardiac impulse originates at the sino-atrial node, and is conducted as a wave over the atria. This wave activates the atrio-ventricular node, and is then transmitted to the ventricles via the Bundle of His and bundle branches. The left bundle perforates the inter-ventricular septum, and depolarizes it from left to right. The Purkinje fibres carry the impulse over the entire endocardial surface of the ventricles, and depolarization takes place from endocardium through the myocardium to the epicardium. The electrical forces generated within the heart travel in multiple directions simultaneously. The electrocardiogram is designed to detect and record these electrical forces graphically, and the generated waveform has been labelled as *P,Q,R,S* and *T* waves. The *P* wave represents atrial depolarization, and the *QRS* complex represents ventricular depolarization. Ventricular repolarization is represented by the *T* wave. Atrial repolarization (*Ta*) cannot normally be seen because the *Ta* wave is usually buried within the *QRS* complex.

These signals are amplified, and (by convention) the display is arranged such that impulses moving towards a surface electrode give rise to an upward (positive) deflection, whilst impulses moving away from the same electrode will be downward (negative).

To help interpret the patterns of electrical movement, electrocardiography is carried out in different planes. When a standard 12 lead electrocardiogram is recorded, the limb leads are normally recorded from the right arm (RA), left arm (LA) and left leg (LL). A fourth lead is traditionally placed on the right leg (RL) which does not record impulses, but serves as a ground (earth) electrode. An equilateral electrical triangle (the Einthoven triangle) is formed by these three planes with the heart in the centre (Figure 3.1). The difference in electrical forces between each pair of electrodes is recorded, and displayed as traces designated the 'standard leads' as originally described by Einthoven. Lead I (LA positive, RA negative) produces an axis that runs from shoulder to shoulder, lead II (LL

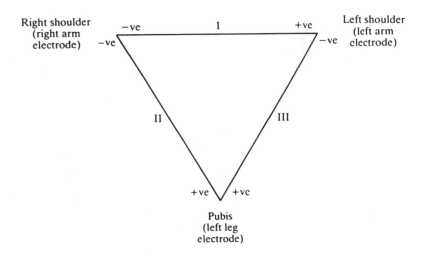

Figure 3.1 The Einthoven triangle (From Jowett and Thompson: Comprehensive Coronary Care (2nd Ed) 1995. Reproduced by kind permission of Academic Press Ltd London)

positive, RA negative) has an axis which runs from the right shoulder
to the left leg, and lead III (LL positive, LA negative) produces an
axis from the left shoulder to the left leg.

In order to help with patient mobility and reduce movement
interference, the bedside ECG is recorded by three or more chest
electrodes. A three lead hook-up traditionally places the electrodes
in the two infra-clavicular spaces (left = positive, right = negative)
with the ground electrode in the 6th intercostal space, in the mid-
clavicular line (Figure 3.2). Whilst this pattern of leads is useful for
most purposes, the goals of electrocardiographic monitoring have
become more complex and involve components other than simple
dysrhythmia recognition. Furthermore, the ground lead often gets
in the way during routine 12 lead ECG recording and prevents
positioning of defibrillator paddles, should they be required.
Moving the ground (leg) electrode to the right side of the chest is
preferable. Other lead arrangements may be more reliable, and
can help explore the precise nature of any rhythm disturbance, eg.
correctly diagnosing broad complex tachycardias. *ST* segment
monitoring is another main indication for electrocardiographic
monitoring which may be useful in patients with unstable angina
or following percutaneous transluminal coronary angioplasty
(PTCA).

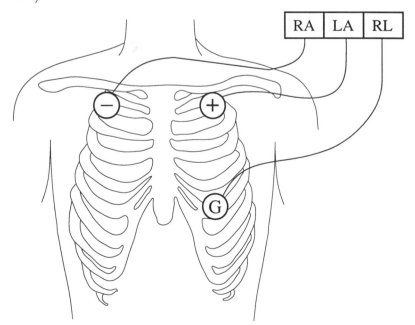

Figure 3.2 Position of the chest electrodes

Interpreting the Waveform

The sinus rhythm ECG waveform is shown in Figure 3.3, and has the following components:

a) The P wave

The normal *P* wave results from the spread of electrical activity from the sino-atrial node across the atria. The *P* wave will be upright in the standard monitor leads. They are not seen in atrial flutter or atrial fibrillation, and may be lost in the *QRS* complex during nodal rhythm. Inverted *P* waves indicate that the atria have been depolarized from an unusual site, and not the sinus node.

b) PR interval

This interval represents the total time taken for the atria to be activated and passage of the impulse through the AV node. The *PR* interval is measured from the start of *P* wave to the beginning of the *QRS* complex. It varies from 0.12–0.20 seconds, shorter intervals being seen at faster heart rates.

A shortened *PR* interval precedes some atrial ectopic beats, particularly if the impulse originates close to the AV junction, or if there are accessory AV conduction pathways (as in Wolff-Parkinson-White syndrome), where a rapidly conducting pathway bypasses the AV node. The *PR* interval is increased if there is atrio-ventricular block caused by drugs or disease (see Chapter 4).

c) QRS complex

The *QRS* duration is measured from the start of the *Q* wave to the end of the *S* wave, and represents the time taken for ventricular depolarization. A value of more than 0.12 seconds is abnormal and usually indicates an intra-ventricular conduction disorder, such as bundle branch block.

The individual components of the *QRS* complex will vary from lead to lead, such that the *R* or *S* wave may be dominant, or the *Q*, *R* or *S* wave may be missing. Exaggerated *QRS* complexes may indicate ventricular hypertrophy. Small *QRS* complexes occur when the heart is 'insulated' from the skin by fat, inflated lungs, or a pericardial effusion.

A pathological *Q* wave has a duration of greater than 0.04 seconds and associates with a variable loss in the height of the following *R* wave (*Q* wave is > 25% of the *R* wave height). *Q* waves normally indicate a previous myocardial infarction.

d) QT interval

This interval represents the time taken from ventricular stimulation to recovery (depolarization and repolarization). It is measured from the beginning of the *QRS* complex to the end of the *T* wave. It normally ranges from 0.35–0.45 seconds, and is very rate sensitive, shortening as the heart rate increases. Correction for the prevailing heart rate to obtain the corrected *QT* interval (*QTc*) may be carried out by applying the formula:

$$QTc = \frac{QT}{\sqrt{RR}}$$

where *QT* is the measured *QT* interval, and *RR* is the time interval between two successive *R* waves (all times in seconds).

For practical purposes, the *QT* interval should be less than 50% of the preceding cycle length (*RR* interval), and seldom exceeds 0.45 seconds. A shortened *QTc* is seen in hyper-calcaemia and hyper-kalaemia. It is prolonged in heart failure, hypo-calcaemia, following myocardial infarction and with certain drugs. Abnormal prolonga-tion of the *QT* interval predisposes to ventricular dysrhythmias, particularly 'torsade de pointes' (see Chapter 5).

e) T wave

The *T* wave results from repolarization of the ventricles and might be assumed to produce a deflection in the opposite direction to the depolarization wave (*QRS* complex). However, repolarization takes place in the opposite direction to depolarization (ie. from epicardium to endocardium), and the *T* wave is usually in the same orientation as the preceding *QRS* complex.

Peaked *T* waves are a feature of hyper-kalaemia, myocardial infarction and ischaemia. Flattening of the *T* wave may occur in hypo-kalaemia. *T* wave inversion may be seen in numerous condi-tions including myocardial infarction, ventricular hypertrophy or with bundle branch block.

f) The ST segment

The *ST* segment is measured from the *J* point (at the junction of the *S* wave and *ST* segment) to the start of the *T* wave. It is usually iso-electric (ie. on the same level as the *PR* segment). Displacement of the *ST* segment both up and down is common, and may accompany myocardial ischaemia or infarction.

g) The U wave

This is a small positive wave which is sometimes seen following the *T* wave. Its cause is unknown. It tends to become exaggerated in hyperkalaemia. Inverted *U* waves are associated with coronary heart disease, which may be a transient feature seen during exercise stress testing, and is often overlooked.

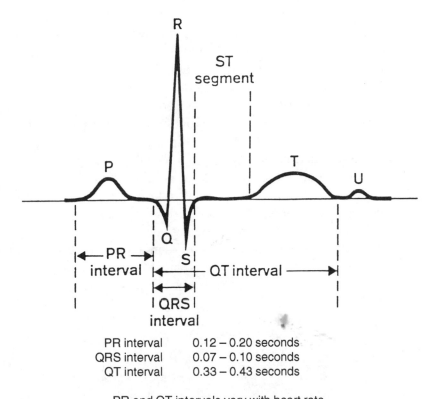

PR interval	0.12 – 0.20 seconds
QRS interval	0.07 – 0.10 seconds
QT interval	0.33 – 0.43 seconds

PR and QT intervals vary with heart rate

Figure 3.3 The sinus rhythm ECG waveform

Electrodes

Electrodes are the small sensors which are fixed to the skin to allow the electrical activity of the heart to be detected and transmitted to the monitor where it is amplified and displayed. Great advances have been made in the design of these simple pieces of equipment and modern disposable, pre-gelled, self-adhesive electrodes usually obtain excellent skin contact with minimal or no skin preparation

(Figure 3.4). Nevertheless, there are several steps which may be taken if the signal is poor:

a)   The skin should be shaved, particularly if the patient is very hairy. Not only will skin contact be enhanced, but the patient will be grateful during electrode removal.

b)   Rubbing the skin with dry gauze or a wooden spatula will remove loose, dry skin and aids electrode contact.

c)   Wiping the skin with alcohol will remove excess tissue debris, body oil and sweat. If the patient is perspiring heavily, a small amount of tincture of benzoin should be applied and allowed to dry before electrode placement.

d)   Check the expiry date of the electrode, and make sure there is a gel-filled sponge on it. Old electrodes may have lost their sponge or have dried out. When in use, the gel soaks into the skin and a period of up to 15 minutes may elapse before good contact is made. Electrode jelly massaged into the skin before application of the electrode will reduce this time. The electrodes should be applied 'centre-first', so that the adhesive holds the gelled area tightly to the skin.

e)   Check that all the electrodes are identical. Using more than one type of electrode on the same patient may distort the trace, since the electrical resistance differs between different makes.

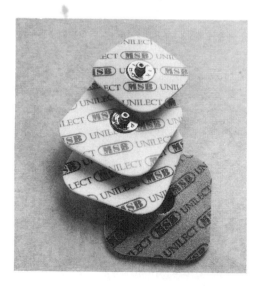

Figure 3.4 Chest electrodes (Reproduced by kind permission of MSB Ltd, Wiltshire)

The electrode site should be examined daily for allergic skin reactions, but otherwise there is no need to change the electrodes routinely unless the signal becomes poor. Patients who are sweating freely may require frequent electrode changes and special super-adhesive electrodes have been manufactured for these patients. Non-allergenic electrodes may be used if the patient is sensitive to the adhesive, and any inflammation may be treated with a small quantity of 1% hydrocortisone cream.

The admitting nurse usually selects the appropriate lead placement for the individual patient before electrode application. If the patient is already on a monitor, it should not be assumed that electrode placement is correct or satisfactory. Proper fixation and cable attachment should be checked at the start of each nursing shift. Once confirmed, documentation of the lead being monitored should be made in the notes and on any rhythm strip which is obtained.

The Monitor Cable

The signals detected by the electrodes are transmitted to the oscilloscope by a monitor cable. At the patient end, this comprises thin wires of about 12 in in length which connect directly to the surface electrodes. The monitor wires either clip or snap onto the chest wires, although it is preferable to do this before the electrodes are placed on the chest. This prevents injuring the patient if firm pressure is required to push them on.

Most electrocardiographic monitoring is undertaken by a three lead hook-up comprising a positive electrode, a negative electrode and a ground (earth) electrode. The junction box on the connecting cable usually has connectors labelled as right arm ('RA' or 'right'), left arm ('LA' or 'left') and right or left leg ('RL', 'LL', 'foot' or 'ground' or 'earth'). Colour coding may also be utilised to differentiate the different leads, but caution is required as there are different colour coding systems. The most common colours are red (RA), yellow (LA) and black or green (RL/LL). These are attached to electrodes placed under the right clavicle (RA), under the left clavicle (LA) and over the lower left chest (RL/LL), in a 'traffic light' sequence involving the clockwise attachment of red, yellow and green leads.

The standard leads are bipolar and record the potential difference between just two electrodes, with the third serving only as an earth (or ground). When recording the electrocardiogram, the basic three electrode bipolar chest lead system produce standard leads I, II and III as follows:

	LA	RA	RL/LL
Lead I:	+ve	−ve	G
Lead II:	G	−ve	+ve
Lead III:	−ve	G	+ve

Selection of the required lead does not mean that the connectors have to be moved, but may be facilitated by a switch on the monitor (the lead selector) which automatically adjusts the lead polarity, and allows selection of standard leads I, II and III simply by turning the switch. Some cables may allow for a further one or two surface electrodes to be attached (four or five electrode hook-up). The four electrode hook-up requires a second leg electrode (placed over the lower right chest), and enables the augmented leads aVR, aVL and aVF to be recorded. The five electrode hook-up adds an exploring chest electrode to allow modified chest leads V1–V6 to be obtained (the MCL leads) in addition to the six standard leads.

The contacts with the electrodes should be clean, and compatible with the surface electrodes being used. The wires should be inspected for bends, knots or breaks in the insulation. It is useful to form a 'stress loop' with this part of the cable to prevent traction on the electrodes and monitor connections, with consequent electrode separation and movement artifact. A lead-fault indicator signal may be present on the monitor, which alerts the nurse to problems in signal transmission.

The monitor cable plugs directly into the bedside monitor, and should be flexible and long enough to allow the patient to walk around the bed area and make use of the commode.

The Bedside Monitor

A bedside monitor is an oscilloscope connected to the patient by the monitor cable which displays the ECG tracing on a continuous basis. Most have non-fade screens which keep the ECG pattern visible across the screen. Where there is a central monitoring system with a central console, the ECG pattern is duplicated for all monitored beds.

The heart rate is usually calculated by a computer which senses the interval between the tallest component of the complexes (usually the R waves). False heart rates may be registered if, for example, the T wave is of equal amplitude to the R wave, since this will be read as another *QRS* complex. The height of these complexes may be adjusted by using the gain control, or if this is insufficient, another lead should be selected by the operating the lead selector control. The rate alarm should be set at 10–15 beats above and below the rates estimated as acceptable for each individual patient.

Many bedside units have a secondary ECG trace under the actual 'real-time' trace. This may run continually, but be delayed so that the trace can be frozen to capture rhythm disturbances by use of the 'run/hold' switch. Depending upon the degree of sophistication, the memory loop will hold a few seconds of the preceding ECG for several minutes. It may allow specific rhythm retrieval and a 'hard copy' rhythm strip to be obtained for more detailed examination, or to provide a permanent copy for the patient's records.

The ECG tracing should be observed for the quality of the recording. Monitoring is usually at 25 mm/second. If the machine is set at 50 mm/second, the rate appears slowed and intervals prolonged. The tracing should be clear, well defined and should travel across the screen at the same level. With routine ECG monitoring, the shape of the *QRS* complexes is often not important, since it is the cardiac rhythm which is usually being assessed. However, advanced electrocoronary monitoring techniques are often undertaken on coronary care units during thrombolysis, or on intensive care units following coronary re-vascularisation procedures, which are used to detect unstable ischaemia, or more precisely define the cardiac rhythm. In these cases, the precise *QRS* morphology and *ST* segment position may be of greater importance (see below).

Monitoring faults are not uncommon. These include:

a) Problems with the trace

If the trace does not appear, all connections should be checked, and the brightness switch should be turned up. If a telemetry unit, the batteries should be checked. The trace position switch may been set such that the trace is off the screen and should be adjusted if required. The 'run/hold' switch should also be activated. The gain control may need adjusting to produce a big enough complex. The minimum brightness should be selected on the contrast control to prevent a 'halo' effect around the tracing.

b) Incorrect heart rate display

The heart rate is normally shown on the rate-meter which counts successive *R* waves, and calculates the heart rate per minute. The system is not infallible. If the *R* wave is too small, or varying in height, it will not be counted. It is also important to ensure that the *T* wave is not too large, or it may be counted and analysed as an extra *QRS* complex. As a result, a doubled heart rate will be displayed.

c) Wandering baseline

Normal respiration or changes in the patient's position in bed may effect the height of the complexes, or give rise to a wandering baseline. The electrodes should be checked, and any excessive cable movement reduced. If there is no improvement, the chest electrodes should be moved, or a different lead selected by the lead selector control.

d) Artifacts and interference

The most frequent problem of static monitoring is false alarms due to movement artifact or loose and poorly connected electrodes. Very small or 'fuzzy' complexes may result on the screen, or even the appearances of asystole. Sixty-cycle interference may be present if the bed or other nearby equipment is not earthed. Similarly, electrical equipment close to the monitor, such as X-ray machines, vacuum pumps, fluorescent lights or electric razors may cause interference.

Somatic tremor produces an uneven, tremulous baseline when the electrodes pick up signals from tensed muscles in anxious patients.

e) Low voltage ECGs

Low voltage complexes (< 6mm) may occur in the frontal leads (peripheral low voltage) or in both the frontal and horizontal planes (total low voltage). Causes may be cardiac (pericardial effusion, cardiomyopathy, diffuse ischaemic heart disease) or non-cardiac (obesity, emphysema, hypo-thyroidism), or both. It may be necessary to re-site or replace the electrodes. The gain control may need turning up.

f) Inappropriate setting of the gain control

Proper setting of the gain control is essential for quality monitoring. If turned up too high, not only will the monitor lead to double counting as described above, but the top of the *QRS* complex will be 'clipped', and may distort the *QRS* morphology which may be important for correct diagnosis. Undersetting the gain control may abolish the *P* wave complex, and may also lead to under-counting the heart rate with inappropriate setting off of the alarms.

The monitor should be placed in good view. Traditionally, monitors are placed on the patient's bedside table to become camouflaged by fruit, flowers, chocolates and get-well cards! On high dependency units, the monitors are usually mounted high on the wall which keeps them out of the way, and easily seen. On general wards they should be placed on a separate, clearly visible table. Nurses should take time to inform the patient and relatives that although the heart is being monitored, it does not necessarily mean that he or she is critically ill. The patient must always be checked each time an alarm sounds to determine validity, particularly on units with separate cubicles. The patient and any visitors should receive an explanation if the alarm sounds.

Positioning the Chest Leads for Advanced ECG Monitoring

The value of electrocardiographic monitoring may be enhanced if consideration is given to the prime purpose of monitoring. Electrode positioning may need modification depending upon whether the aim is to detect ischaemia or dysrhythmia. Chest electrode positioning may need further adjustment if there are problems with rhythm interpretation, as may occur in the diagnosis of recurrent broad complex tachycardias.

Several modifications to the basic three electrode bipolar chest lead system have been described which enables particular areas of the heart to be looked at more closely. If the three standard leads are connected together through high resistance, they form a common 'central' terminal of zero potential. If this is then used as an indifferent terminal, another active electrode can be used to explore the rest of the heart. This is the basis of the unipolar lead system in normal 12 lead electrocardiography. A modified bipolar lead system has been developed because static monitoring normally employs just three electrodes, whilst a true unipolar system would require five electrodes.

The modified three electrode bipolar system designates the negative electrode as 'central' (denoted by the letter 'C'), followed by a letter indicating which electrode is being modified to become central. For example, the abbreviation CL means that the left arm electrode has been designated the 'C' lead (ie. C = LA = negative or indifferent electrode). Similarly, leads described as CR and CF indicate that the negative electrode are the right arm and left leg, respectively. The letter M is used in front of these letters to show that the position has been modified. For example, in MCL leads the central lead has been modified by moving it down from the left arm to the left infra-clavicular space. Finally, a number is used to signify the position of the positive (or exploring) electrode on the chest, according to the normal pre-cordial V lead positions (V1–V6). For example, in MCL-1, the negative electrode (C) has been modified by moving it from its normal position below the right clavicle to below the left clavicle (ie. MCL), and the positive electrode is placed in the position of chest lead V1.

The MCL Leads

The MCL lead system enables all the standard pre-cordial chest (V) leads to be simulated by placing the negative lead under the left clavicle, and placing the positive in the usual pre-cordial position for V1 to V6. Such leads are then designated MCL-1 to MCL-6. MCL-1 is the lead of choice if only single-channel monitoring is available, whilst MCL-1 and MCL-6 are frequently used together in dual-channel monitoring.

1) MCL-1 (Modified Lead V1)

Electrode positions: The positive (RL/LL) electrode is placed in the normal V1 chest lead position (4th right intercostal space), whilst the negative and the ground electrodes are located near the left shoulder (LA) and right shoulder (RA) respectively (Figure 3.5). The posterior aspect of the shoulders may be utilised rather than the infra-clavicular spaces to keep the leads out of the way.

Lead III should be selected on the monitor so that the left leg lead becomes the positive (exploring) lead.

Uses: MCL-1 clearly demonstrates the P wave, and usually allows differentiation between ventricular ectopic beats and aberrantly conducted supra-ventricular beat (ie. beats conducted to the ventricles with bundle branch block). Aberration should be expected when the ectopic beat is preceded by a P wave different from that of a normal sinus beat, or if it is a right bundle branch block pattern ('M' shaped rather than 'W' shaped).

MCL-1 is also useful for diagnosing bundle branch block, and for differentiating between left and right ventricular ectopic beats. In right bundle branch block, the left ventricle is depolarized before the right, and the net electrical movement is towards the V1 electrode, producing a predominantly positive complex. This pattern should also be seen in an ectopic beat arising from the left ventricle. In left bundle branch block and with right ventricular ectopic beats however, the converse applies with the right ventricle being depolarized before the left. A predominantly negative V1 complex is then recorded by the MCL-1 electrode.

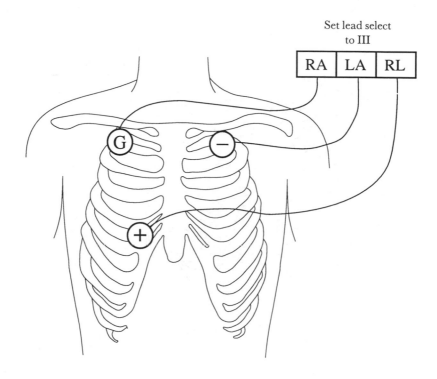

Set lead select
to III

| RA | LA | RL |

Figure 3.5 MCL-1

2) MCL-6 (Modified lead V6)

Electrode positions: The negative and ground electrodes are kept in the same position as for MCL-1, but the positive (exploring) electrode is moved to the 5th intercostal space in the mid-axillary line (V6) position (Figure 3.6). The lead selector must remain on 'lead III'.

Uses: Like MCL-1, MCL-6 is also useful for differentiating right and left bundle branch block and differentiating ventricular ectopic beats from aberrantly conducted supra-ventricular beats. *P* waves are not so clear. MCL-6 is useful for patients where the right precordial lead of MCL-1 is impracticable (eg. following cardiac surgery), or in patients with barrel chests (eg. patients with chronic bronchitis) where MCL-1 recordings are often associated with poor signals.

Other Modified Leads

1) MCR leads

Electrode positions: Lead *MCR-1* is modified by placing the negative (RA) electrode under the right clavicle, the positive (LA) electrode is

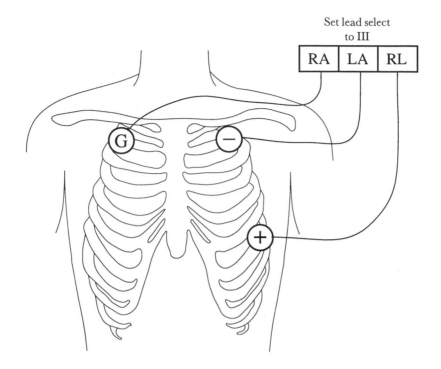

Figure 3.6 MCL-6

placed in the chest lead V1 position with the ground electrode in the usual LL/RL position (Figure 3.7).

Uses: The MCR leads are useful for *P* wave demonstration. Sometimes, the *P* wave may be better visualised by placing the precordial electrode in the third right interspace (MCR-3), or even further round the right chest (MCR-4−MCR-6).

Lead *MCR-5* is sometimes known as CS-5 (central sub-clavicular lead) and is excellent for detecting anterior ischaemia either during stress testing or in the operating theatre. Switching the lead selector from lead I to lead II changes the monitoring lead to standard lead II since the LL/RL electrode is in the right position (it will become positive), and allows the inferior aspect of the heart to be monitored both for rhythm and ischaemia (Figure 3.8).

2) M3

Electrode positions: The shoulder electrode positions are similar to MCL-6, but the positive electrode (RL/LL) is moved from the V6 chest position to the right upper abdomen (Figure 3.9). Lead III is selected on the monitor switch.

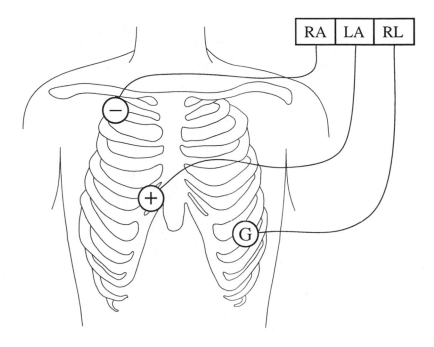

Figure 3.7 MCR-1

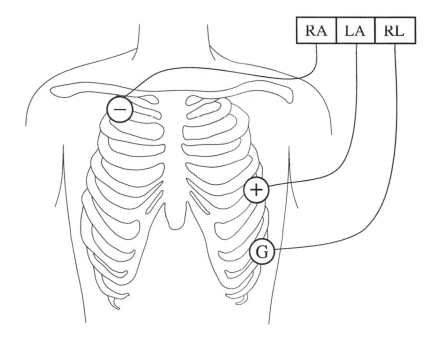

Figure 3.8 CS5

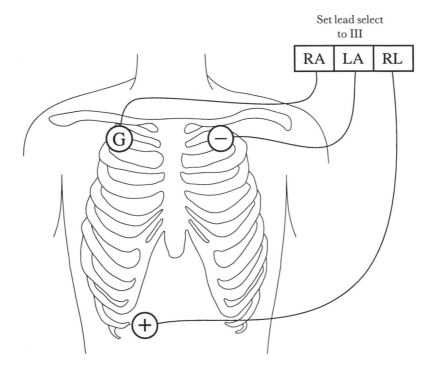

Figure 3.9 M3

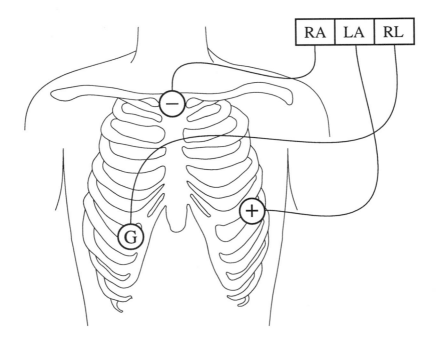

Figure 3.10 CM5

Uses: This lead is of particular value is determining retrograde *P* waves.

3) CM5 (Central manubrium lead V5)

Electrode positions: The negative (RA) electrode is placed over the upper sternum (the manubrium), the positive (LA) electrode is in the V5 chest position with the ground placed over the lower right chest (Figure 3.10).

Uses: CM5 is useful for detecting anterior ischaemic *ST* segment changes and evidence of left ventricular strain.

4) CB5 (Central back lead V5)

Electrode positions: The negative (RA) electrode is placed over the centre of the right scapula, the positive (LA) electrode is placed in the V5 chest position with the ground (RL/LL) in its usual position (Figure 3.11).

Uses: CB5 shows good *P* wave morphology (since it lies close to the right atrium), and ischaemic *ST* segment changes (like pre-cordial lead V5). It is therefore very useful for patients with cardiac disease who are undergoing surgery and need peri-operative monitoring.

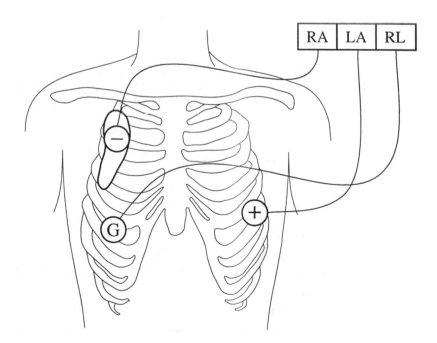

Figure 3.11 CB5

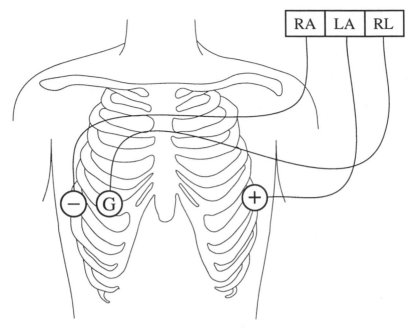

Figure 3.12 CC5

5) CC5 (Chest chest lead V5)

Electrode positions: The negative (RA) electrode is placed in the right anterior axillary line in the 5th rib interspace, the positive electrode is placed in the chest V5 position with the ground (LL/RL) in its usual place (Figure 3.12).

Uses: This is another good lead for monitoring for ischaemia.
A summary of the lead positions, polarity and lead selector switch is shown in Table 3.1.

Choice of Lead Arrangements

There are three common clinical circumstances which affect choice of lead arrangement:

1) Following acute myocardial infarction

For monitoring following acute myocardial infarction, the most useful lead systems are MCL-1 and M3. This is because the electrode positions do not cover the apex of the heart which must remain exposed to allow auscultation and defibrillation, if required. In addition, these configurations can be used to maximise information about dysrhythmia.

2) During unstable ischaemia, or where it may occur (eg. unstable angina, following coronary angioplasty or thrombolysis).

Following re-cannalisation of coronary arteries, either by thrombolytic therapy or percutaneous transluminal coronary angioplasty (PTCA), there is a period of instability during which re-occlusion may take place. Clearly, the sooner this complication is recognised the better, so that further treatment may be instituted to re-open the coronary artery. For reasons which are not clear, re-occlusion is not always symptomatic, and may thus go unrecognised unless the ECG is being monitored specifically for *ST* segment changes. Whether there is *ST* elevation or *ST* depression is usually not important, but detection of *ST* segment shift may be missed if monitoring is by inappropriate leads.

The most sensitive leads for detecting *ST* segment shift depend upon the area of ischaemia:

a)   For the left anterior descending coronary artery

Modified antero-septal chest leads V2, V3 and V4 (MCL-2, MCL-3 and MCL-4)

b)   For the left circumflex artery

Modified lateral leads V5 and V6 (MCL-5, MCL-6) and aVL

c)   For the right coronary artery

Inferior leads II, III and aVF.

Table 3.1: Bipolar Lead Selection for ECG Monitoring with Three Chest Electrodes (RA, LA, RL/LL)

LEAD	I	II	III	MCL 1	MCL 6	MCR 1	CS5	M3	CM5	CB5	CC5
ELECTRODE											
RA	−ve	−ve	G	G	G	−ve	−ve	G	−ve	−ve	−ve
LA	+ve	G	−ve	−ve	−ve	+ve	+ve	−ve	+ve	+ve	+ve
RL	G	+ve	+ve	+ve	+ve	G	G	+ve	G	G	G
Selector Switch Position	I	II	III	III	III	I	I	III	I	I	I

Key
+ve = positive electrode
−ve = negative electrode
G = ground or earth electrode
See text for positioning of skin electrodes

3) Episodic broad complex tachycardia of uncertain origin

Recording MCL-1 is essential when monitoring for broad complex tachycardia, and MCL-6 may be required as well. Lead MCL-1 recordings may help distinguish between ventricular and supra-ventricular tachycardia if the *QRS* complex is positive in MCL-1 (Figure 3.13). Ventricular tachycardia will show a broad *QRS* complex with a dominant primary *R* wave in the *RSR* complex (ie. the left rabbit's ear is longer – *Rsr*). The *QRS* pattern in aberrantly conducted supra-ventricular tachycardia will appear broad, but the secondary *R* wave will be dominant (the right rabbit's ear is longer – *rSR*). If the *QRS* is negative in MCL-1, MCL-6 is required to see if there is concordance (as in ventricular tachycardia), and a lead which shows the *P* waves accurately (eg. MCR-3) may be vital in demonstrating AV dissociation. The various ways of diagnosing broad complex tachycardias is described further in Chapter 5.

Because patients with unstable ischaemia are also at risk of dysrhythmias, the placement of leads requires careful consideration to maximise information about ischaemia and dysrhythmia. If dual-channel monitoring is available, then MCL-1 should be on one channel, since this is of major value in diagnosing broad complex dysrhythmias. The second channel will depend either on the pre-thrombolytic ECG (which will give some indication of the affected artery), or according to which artery was dilated at PTCA.

When monitoring with a single-channel monitor, the choice must lie between using the best diagnostic lead from a rhythm point of view (usually MCL-1), or a lead which will detect the best *ST*

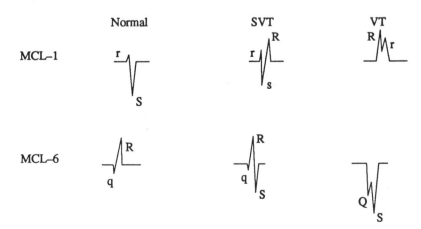

Figure 3.13 Normal MCL-1 and MCL-6 QRS patterns compared to morphology during supra-ventricular tachycardia (SVT) and ventricular tachycardia (VT)

segment shift, according to which coronary artery is likely to be affected. Regardless of this, if re-occlusion is suspected a full 12 lead ECG should always be taken to accurately document *ST* segment shift as evidence of continuing ischaemia.

Multi-channel ECG Monitors

Reference has already been made to bedside monitors which have the capability for recording and displaying two or three channels simultaneously. Monitors should always be used to their full potential by utilising all channels to maximise the information attainable. The mode most often used in dual-channel monitoring is the display of MCL-1 and MCL-6 simultaneously and may be achieved via four surface electrodes. If three ECG channels are available, then the usual choice is standard lead I, aVF and V1. The V1 lead should not need to be modified as MCL-1 if the system has a five lead hook-up, since a 'true' unipolar V1 lead is possible.

Some coronary care units always monitor with a five lead hook-up (two infra-clavicular spaces, lower left chest, lower right chest and one in the V5 position) which allows the selection of any two of seven leads (I, II, III, aVR, aVL, aVF and V5). Leads II and V5 are the usual first choice which enable both inferior and anterior ischaemia to be detected.

Invasive Monitoring

Invasive techniques are sometimes required for precise definition of dysrhythmias. Oesophageal electrocardiography utilises a lead passed into the oesophagus, rather like a naso-gastric tube, and is excellent for recording atrial activity since the lead is placed directly behind the left atrium, which lies adjacent to the oesophagus. The usual naming of the lead is derived from the distance in centimetres from the nose to the electrode. Thus O_{50} positions the electrode 50 centimetres from the tip of the nose. Lead O_{15-25} will be positioned approximately behind the left atrium, and O_{40-50} should lie behind the left ventricle. Precise localisation, however, may require fluoroscopy. Until recently, the technique was not widely used because of patient discomfort associated with placement of the naso-gastric tube. Now, an easily swallowed, gel-covered 'pill' electrode can be used by cooperative patients for both short-term and 24 hour ambulatory monitoring with no or little discomfort. The gelatine capsule dissolves leaving the exposed electrode.

The oesophageal electrode has particular use in differentiating atrial flutter from atrial fibrillation and sinus tachycardia, and exploring the posterior surface of the left ventricle.

The use of intra-cardiac electrodes may help to determine atrio-ventricular activation sequences. Electrodes positioned in the region of the tricuspid valve and right ventricle may then be used to record electrical potentials in the Bundle of His. These specialised techniques are of particular value in differentiating supra-ventricular from ventricular dysrhythmias, and in the identification of accessory pathways and the site of block in atrio-ventricular conduction defects.

Telemetry

Monitoring by telemetry allows early mobilisation of the patient without losing the advantage of continuous ECG monitoring. The chest electrodes are positioned:

> LA = under the left clavicle (+ve)
> RA = under the right clavicle (–ve)
> RL = right sternal edge (ground)

The chest leads are attached to a small portable radio-transmitter which relays the hearts electrical activity to the central console using radio waves rather than a monitor cable (Figure 3.14). Reproduction of the ECG is usually not so reliable, since patient movement and physical structures may interfere with transmission and reception of the waveform.

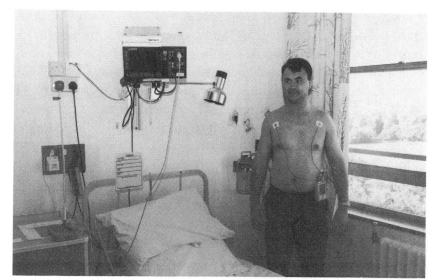

Figure 3.14 A telemetry unit

Signal-averaged electrocardiagraphy

This technique allows identification of low voltage signals at the end of the *QRS* complex ('late potentials') whose presence associates with ventricular dysrhythmias, and may thus help in prognostic assessment following acute myocardial infarction. A large number of *QRS* complexes are recorded, superimposed and filtered electronically, and the low voltage signal amplified. Recording signal averaged ECGs requires specialised equipment. The detection of late potentials may be of prognostic significance in patients with cardiac disease.

Interpretation of the Dysrhythmias

Dysrhythmias may be recognised on the monitor, but are often best printed out on ECG paper for detailed analysis and storage. Standard ECG graph paper is made up of horizontal and vertical lines at one millimetre intervals (Figure 3.15). A heavier line is present every 5 mm. The vertical lines are time markers, with each faint line being equivalent to 0.04 of a second, and each darker line being 0.2 seconds. The horizontal lines determine voltage measured upwards or downwards from the iso-electric line. The iso-electric line is taken as the flat line between the *T* and the *P* wave. Movement above this line is termed a positive deflection, and movement below it termed a negative deflection. The ECG is recorded at 25 mm/second with a usual calibration of 1 mV = 10 mm.

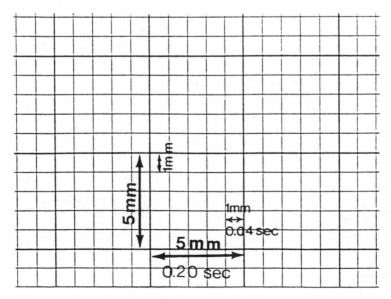

Figure 3.15 Standard ECG paper

It is good practice to adopt a systematic approach to rhythm analysis so that false interpretations are not made.

a) Calculation of the heart rate

The rate-meter on the ECG monitor will usually give an accurate recording of the heart rate. This may be checked on the rhythm strip by dividing 300 by the number of large ECG squares between successive *R* waves. If the rhythm is irregular, it is better to count the number of *R* waves on a 6 second strip and multiply by 10 to obtain the heart rate. The top of the ECG is usually marked automatically in 3 second intervals. 'ECG rulers' have been specifically designed to measure the heart rate and other *PQRST* intervals.

b) Assessing regularity

A regular heart rate is usually obvious on simple inspection. *R* wave regularity may easily be checked by marking them on a plain piece of paper held adjacent to the trace. Moving the plain paper in either direction should not interrupt the match of marks and *R* waves. There may be a slight irregularity with breathing (sinus arrhythmia), but the *R–R* intervals should not differ by more than 0.12 seconds.

c) Look for P waves

If *P* waves occur regularly, are of normal shape and precede every *QRS* complex, sinus rhythm is present. Absent or malformed *P* waves imply impulse formation outside the SA node.

d) Measure the PR interval

This should be between 0.1–0.2 seconds.

e) Measure the QRS interval

This should not be longer than 0.12 seconds.

f) Observe for any extra or additional ECG changes

The dysrhythmias are described in the next two chapters as follows:

Rate
Rhythm
P Waves
PR Interval
QRS Complex
Remarks
Aetiology

It is hoped that the bedside monitor will display *normal sinus rhythm*, which is characterised by:

Rate: 60–100 beats per minute
Rhythm: Regular
P Waves: Regularly precede each *QRS* complex and are upright
PR Interval: 0.12–0.20 seconds
QRS Complex: Narrow (< 0.12 seconds)

Remarks: The *PR* and *QT* interval vary with heart rate, becoming shorter as the heart rate increases.
Minor changes in an otherwise regular pattern may be caused by a *sinus arrhythmia* (Figure 3.16).

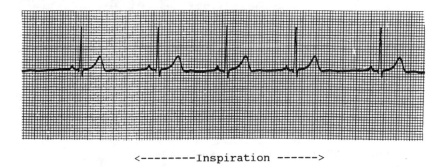

<-------Inspiration ------>

Figure 3.16 Sinus arrhythmia. The pulse rate quickens on inspiration, and the R waves become closer together

Aetiology: A sinus arrhythmia is seen commonly in young individuals, when an increase in heart rate is seen during inspiration, and a slowing during expiration. It is a normal response to increased cardiac filling when an increased negative intra-thoracic pressure occurs during inspiration causes the venous return to increase. The heart rate then quickens to eject the increased load.

Chapter 4
Slow Heart
Rhythms

Slow heart rates are known as bradycardias and predispose to ventricular standstill. *Pseudo-bradycardias* may be caused by alternate or multiple regular ectopic beats, such that only sinus beats are appreciated when taking the radial pulse. An electrocardiogram (ECG) will demonstrate all the complexes and show that this is not a true bradycardia.

True bradycardias occur either as a result of:

Sino-atrial dysfunction, when generation of the impulse at the sino-atrial (SA) node is inhibited or fails to reach the atria,
   or
Heart block, when conduction of the impulse through the heart is slowed or blocked.

Escape rhythms

The inherent ability of specialised cardiac tissue to initiate electrical impulses is known as automaticity, and the responsible cells are known as pacemaker or automatic cells. In the sino-atrial node, these will discharge spontaneously at about 80 times per minute, but elsewhere automatic cells have a slower discharge rate. For example, in the atrio-ventricular (AV) node, this may be at about 60 times per minute, and within the ventricles the spontaneous discharge rate falls to about 30 times per minute. This back-up system of 'escape rhythms' exists to prevent rhythm failure should the SA node fail to discharge. In this instance, an alternative pacemaker usually takes over, and although the rate will initially be slow, there is a tendency for the rate of this abnormal pacemaker to speed up because of 'enhanced automaticity'. When an ectopic site takes over pacemaker function, and is denoted by the prefix 'idio', for example, idio-nodal tachycardia or idio-ventricular rhythm.

Vagotonic block may occur when there is high vagal tone such as may occur during sleep when sympathetic tone is normally decreased, and vagal stimulation becomes dominant. As a result there may be a sinus bradycardia, sinus pauses or atrio-ventricular conduction block. This phenomenon may be normal (particularly in athletes), but clinically most often occurs following acute inferior myocardial infarction. It may otherwise be induced by drugs (eg. beta-blockers), during endo-tracheal suction or intubation, and occasionally during swallowing or prolonged coughing.

Carotid Sinus Hypersensitivity and the Vasovagal Syndrome

Both these conditions are associated with dizziness and syncope caused by inappropriate vagal overactivity which results in bradycardia and sinus pauses, sometimes in association with a fall in peripheral vascular resistance. Pre-syncope is therefore due to bradycardia or hypotension, or sometimes both.

a) Carotid sinus hypersensitivity

Pre-syncope is associated with sudden head movements, particularly in association with high collars or ties. Sometimes there is no obvious trigger. Artificial carotid sinus massage may demonstrate this hypersensitivity by producing symptoms accompanied by sinus pauses of up to three seconds, or a profound bradycardia.

b) Vasovagal syndrome

This typically occurs in response to stress or emotion when the individual is standing still, although sometimes there is no clear cut trigger. Some patients are found to have an autonomic defect, and the condition is termed 'the malignant vasovagal syndrome'.

Tilt-table testing is generally used for diagnosis, when different degrees of foot down tilt (at 40–80 degrees from the horizontal) are maintained for up to an hour whilst monitoring the ECG and blood pressure. Pre-syncope typically appears in 10–20 minutes associated with bradycardia and hypotension, which recover as soon as the table is returned to the horizontal.

Bradycardias Caused by Sino-atrial Dysfunction

Sino-atrial (SA) dysfunction may lead to sinus bradycardia, sino-atrial block, sinus arrest or junctional escape rhythms. Sometimes the only indication of SA dysfunction is an inability of the heart rate to increase with exercise.

1. Sinus Bradycardia (Figure 4.1)

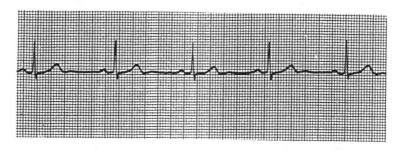

Figure 4.1 Sinus bradycardia

Rate: Less than 60 beats per minute
Rhythm: Regular
P Waves: Normal
PR Interval: Normal
QRS Complex: Normal

Remarks: Sinus bradycardia is arbitrarily defined as a sinus rhythm slower than 60 beats/minute, and although many normal healthy adults will have heart rates below this limit, it is wise to assume that rates of less than 50 beats per minute are abnormal. Bradycardia occurs in about 30% of patients following acute myocardial infarction, and normally indicates parasympathetic over-activity from autonomic fibres supplying the atria and the atrio-ventricular (AV) node. Because afferent vagal fibres are more common on the inferior surface of the heart, inferior ischaemia or infarction is frequently accompanied by vagal over-activity which results in an induced bradycardia. Whilst slowing of the heart is useful to limit myocardial work and thus protect the injured heart, extreme bradycardia may reduce coronary perfusion and lead to hypotension secondary to a reduced cardiac output. Any escape rhythms which occur may predispose to ventricular tachycardia and fibrillation.

Symptoms of sinus bradycardia are uncommon, but sudden onset of any bradycardia may cause dizziness or syncope (Stokes-Adams attacks).

Aetiology: Sinus bradycardia is common in healthy individuals and athletes, especially during sleep (caused by vagotonic block). Other causes of sinus bradycardia include acute myocardial infarction, hypo-thyroidism, raised intra-cranial pressure, infections (eg. acute rheumatic fever, typhoid), sinus node disease, cholestatic jaundice, myocarditis and drugs (especially digoxin, diltiazem, beta-blockers).

A *wandering atrial pacemaker* may be seen when vagal tone is high, causing two supraventricular pacemakers to compete against each other (typically the SA and AV nodes). The site of impulse formation then 'wanders' between these two pacemakers giving rise to *P* waves of varying morphology in association with a variable *PR* interval. The *QRS* complexes are normal as is the heart rate (Figure 4.2). Occasionally, 'wandering' may take place entirely within the SA node, although ECG findings are the same.

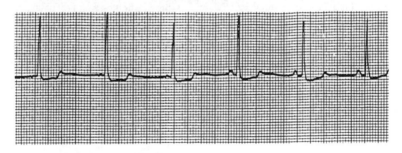

Figure 4.2 Wandering atrial pacemaker

2. Sino-atrial Block

Rate: Slow or normal
Rhythm: Normal with occasional missed beat
P Waves: No *P* wave precedes missed beat
PR Interval: Normal
QRS Complex: A whole *PQRST* complex is dropped

Remarks: Sino-atrial block is said to occur if the sino-atrial node fails to initiate one or more stimuli on time, or if there is block of transmission of the impulse into the atria. The atria and ventricles will not be depolarized and long pauses between successive beats may result.

The blocking of the impulse from the SA node may be classified as type I or type II exit block, but differentiation is sometimes very difficult.

Type I SA exit block occurs when there is progressive delay in transmission of the impulse through the SA node to the atrium, which eventually results in a non-conducted sinus impulse. The *P*–interval becomes progressively longer until a long pause occurs between two beats (so-called 'sino-atrial Wenckebach').

Type II SA exit block occurs when there is abrupt failure of transmission of the SA impulse to the atrium and may be seen in two ways:

a)   Long pauses occur regularly following multiple normal *P–P* cycles. This most often happens every 3–4 beats such that there is little effect on the pulse rate. However, if it occurs with alternate beats, the pulse rate will be halved.

b)   Sinus arrest is characterised by cardiac standstill for varying periods of time (Figure 4.3). Escape beats from the atria, the AV node or the ventricles then takes over pacemaker function.

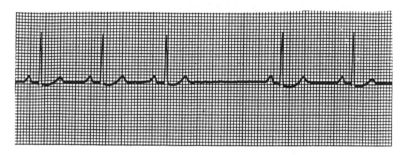

Figure 4.3 Sinus arrest

Aetiology: Since the right coronary artery supplies the SA node in most patients, sino-atrial block is particularly common following acute inferior myocardial infarction, and usually disappears within 48 hours. A similar transient form of SA block may follow DC countershock, especially if the patient is taking drugs which may affect the SA node. Chronic SA block is usually due to idiopathic fibrosis of the node (sick sinus syndrome), although a small proportion are due to chronic myocardial ischaemia. Whilst drugs such as beta-blockers, verapamil, flecainide, amiodarone and methyldopa are usually associated with a sinus bradycardia, they may sometimes be implicated in SA block, particularly if the patient is elderly.

3. Junctional (Nodal) Bradycardia

Rate: 40–60 beats per minute
Rhythm: Regular
P Waves: Abnormal – inverted or occurring before, during or after the *QRS* complex

PR Interval: Shortened
QRS Complex: Normal

Remarks: The AV junction is the second major site of impulse formation. If the SA node fails to initiate an impulse and no other focus
arises in the atria, then the AV junction takes over pacemaker function. This will also happen if the sinus rate falls to a rate approaching
the inherent rate of the AV node (about 50 beats per minute).
AV junctional rhythms are relatively slow at 40–60 beats/minute
(Figure 4.4), but may speed up to produce a relative junctional tachycardia at 60–100 beats/minute (Figure 4.5), or an idio-nodal tachycardia with rates over 100 beats/minute (see Chapter 5). These
dysrhythmias are caused by 'enhanced automaticity' of conduction
tissue and predispose to AV dissociation.

If junctional rhythm is present, the atria and ventricles may be
stimulated at the same time by the nodal pacemaker. The stimulus
passes normally into the ventricles producing a normal *QRS*
complex, but there is also retrograde activation of the atria by the

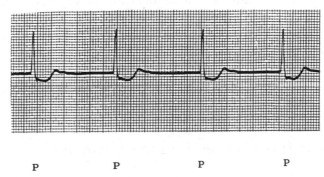

P   P   P   P

Figure 4.4 Junctional rhythm. Note the retrograde P wave at the end of the QRS
complex

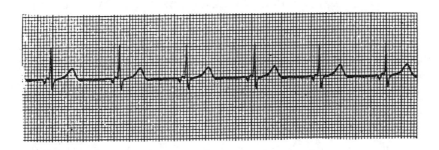

Figure 4.5 Relative nodal (junctional) tachycardia. Note the inverted P waves

same impulse, such that a *P* wave may appear slightly before, slightly after or buried in the *QRS* complex, depending upon the velocity of forward (antegrade) and backward (retrograde) conduction. The retrograde spread of the atrial impulse may be recognised by the shape of the *P* wave which is abnormal and usually inverted in leads II, III and aVF. Reciprocal (echo) beats may occur following a junctional ectopic beat, when the original impulse is conducted slowly in the AV node giving rise to retrograde activation of the atria, followed by a second antegrade beat when the impulse continues around within the AV node to initiate the ventricles a second time.

Because the atria and ventricles are often stimulated together by the nodal impulse spreading proximally and distally at the same time, atrial contraction often takes place against closed mitral and tricuspid valves. Blood is then pumped backwards into the superior vena cava and neck resulting in giant venous *v* waves.

Bradycardias encourage premature ectopic beats which may provide the stimulus for paroxysmal re-entry tachycardias (junctional or ventricular). The bradycardia-tachycardia ('brady-tachy') syndrome is an example of the association of a bradycardia with paroxysmal tachycardias.

Aetiology: Junctional rhythm usually emerges as an escape rhythm following sinus node depression, most often following acute myocardial infarction. It may also be seen in patients with cardiomyopathy, myocarditis or during anaesthesia, particularly if the patient is acidotic or hypoxic.

Bradycardias Caused by Heart Block

Atrio-ventricular Block

Atrio-ventricular block exists when conduction from the atria to the ventricles is either slowed or completely blocked. The conduction disturbance may arise within the atrio-ventricular (AV) node, the Bundle of His or the bundle branches. 'High block' implies the site is in the AV node or the Bundle of His above the bundle branch divisions. 'Low block' implies block below the bundle branch divisions. Inter-His and multi-site blocks can also occur.

Heart block may be transient, intermittent or permanent, and usually results in bradycardia with or without hypotension. Heart block predisposes to ventricular standstill and sudden death.

Dysfunction of the AV node has been classified as first, second or third degree AV block.

a) First degree heart block (Figure 4.6)

Rate: Normal
Rhythm: Regular
P Waves: Normal
PR Interval: Prolonged (> 0.20 seconds)
QRS Complex: Normal

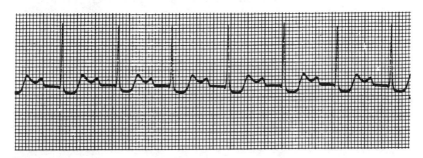

Figure 4.6 First degree heart block

Remarks: First degree heart block indicates a conduction delay between the atria and the ventricles, and is characterised by prolongation of the *PR* interval. The *PR* interval is made up of time taken for intra-atrial conduction (10–50 msec), AV nodal conduction (90–150 msecs) and His-Purkinje conduction (22–55 msec), and the total conduction time is measured on the ECG from the beginning of the *P* wave to the beginning of the *QRS* complex, regardless of whether this is an *R* wave or a *Q* wave. The *PR* interval varies with age, but does not usually exceed 0.2 seconds unless the impulse passing from the atria to the ventricles is delayed at the AV node (or rarely in the atria or Bundle of His). There is no change in heart rate, so that first degree heart block may only be appreciated on the ECG.

Aetiology: First degree AV block may be a normal and benign finding in young adults, but in others may progress to higher degrees of AV blockade. Any cause of increased parasympathetic (vagal) tone can delay AV conduction and prolong the *PR* interval. Transient causes include vomiting, straining and carotid sinus massage. Drugs acting at the AV node, such as digoxin, diltiazem and beta-blockers may also produce first degree heart block. Acute inferior myocardial infarction is a common acute cause of AV block.

b) Second degree heart block

This is a partial atrio-ventricular block which results in some of the atrial impulses failing to reach the ventricles. There are two types of second degree heart block.

i) Mobitz type I (Wenckebach) AV block (Figure 4.7)

Rate: Normal or slow

Rhythm: Irregular due to dropped ventricular complexes

P Waves: Normal morphology but there are more *P* waves than *QRS* complexes

PR Interval: Progressively lengthens with each beat until a dropped beat occurs. The *PR* interval then shortens again and the cycle repeats.

QRS Complex: Normal

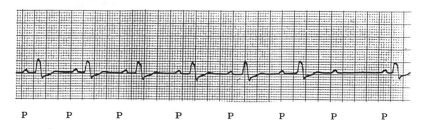

Figure 4.7 Second degree (Mobitz type 1) heart block (Wenckebach). The PR interval gradually increases until a whole QRS is dropped

Remarks: This is the more common form of second degree heart block (90%). Each successive stimulus from the atria finds it more difficult to pass through the AV junction, reflected as a progressive prolongation of the *PR* interval recorded on the ECG. Eventually, the stimulus is unable to pass through to the ventricles, and the atrial *P* wave is not followed by a *QRS* complex. When the next atrial impulse arrives at the AV junction, it is able to pass through normally since the tissues have recovered, and the cycle then repeats. The overall appearance of the rhythm is of 'group beating'. That is, groups of complexes separated by a pause. The frequency of dropped beats varies and may be numerous or very few.

ii) Mobitz type II AV block (Figure 4.8)

Rate: Usually slow at half, third or quarter the atrial rate

Rhythm: Usually regular

P Waves: Two or more per *QRS* complex

PR Interval: Constant in conducted beats

QRS Complex: Normal or may be widened as there is sometimes coexistent bundle branch block

Remarks: During type II AV block, the AV junction does not respond to every atrial stimulus and the observed rhythm often called 2:1 or 4:1 heart block, to denote the ratio of atrial to ventricular

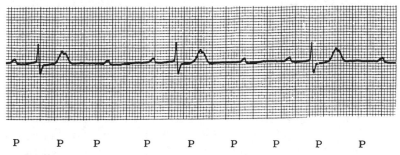

P   P   P   P   P   P   P   P   P

Figure 4.8 Second degree heart block (Mobitz type II)

beats. The *PR* interval is constant in conducted beats, and the pulse is regular. The *QRS* complex is often widened because of simultaneous blockade of the bundle branches. This form of AV block is usually more serious, being associated with slow ventricular rates, Stokes-Adams attacks and sudden death.

Aetiology: For a long time it was thought that the site of blockade within the conduction pathway was high in Mobitz type 1 and low in Mobitz type II, and that prognosis was often good for the former and poor for the latter. However, electrophysiological and histological studies have shown that the distinction is not clear cut. There is no doubt that the Wenckebach phenomenon is often benign, particularly if observed during sleep. It may also be functional (eg. during supraventricular tachycardias), or due to electrolyte imbalance or drugs which suppress AV conduction, such as digoxin, diltiazem, etc. However, its significance in those with myocardial disease is not necessarily so benign, and that is particularly so with Mobitz type II heart block which frequently associates with severe myocardial disease.

c) Third degree (complete) heart block (Figure 4.9)

Rate: Ventricular rate 30–40 beats per minute. Atrial rate is faster at 60–100 beats per minute

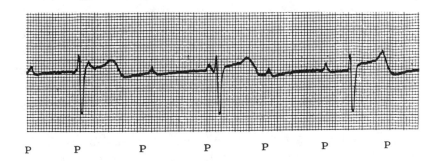

P   P   P   P   P   P   P

Figure 4.9 Third degree (complete) heart block

Rhythm: Regular or irregular
P Waves: Normal and unrelated to *QRS* complexes
PR Interval: Never constant
QRS Complex: Slightly or considerably widened, depending upon the site of the secondary pacemaker

Remarks: In complete heart block, transmission of atrial impulses through to the ventricles are totally blocked, either at or below the AV junction. Ventricular activity can only be maintained by an escape rhythm which takes over from within the distal AV node, the His-Purkinje system or the ventricles. *P* waves occur regularly but have no relationship to the slower ventricular *QRS* complexes. If complete heart block occurs with atrial fibrillation, there are no *P* waves and complete heart block can only be recognised by appreciation of the ectopic ventricular pacemaker which will be slow and with abnormal *QRS* morphology.

The heart rate and *QRS* morphology will vary during complete heart block, depending upon the origin of the secondary pacemaker. If the block is high, the *QRS* complex is usually normal unless there is a coexistent bundle branch block. However, if the block is low, the ectopic pacemaker usually arises in either the left or right bundle producing a widened *QRS* complex at a slower rate. In general, the lower down the conducting system that the secondary pacemaker arises, the slower the rate, the wider the complex and the higher the associated mortality. The lowest pacemakers are often very irregular with a propensity to interposed ventricular ectopic beats and ventricular standstill.

Aetiology: The atrio-ventricular node may be affected by myocarditis, collagen disorders or by drugs, such as digoxin, diltiazem and beta-adrenergic blocking agents. Fibrosis of the AV junction is probably the most common cause of chronic complete heart block, particularly in elderly men. Certain infections may cause a transient heart block such as rheumatic fever, viral myo-pericarditis and endocarditis. Sometimes, complete heart block only occurs during exercise, and may cause syncope or weakness during exertion.

Acute heart block occurs in the early phase of 10% of cases of acute myocardial infarction. With inferior infarction, the pacemaker is usually high nodal and often develops slowly following first and second degree heart block. The rate is usually regular and haemodynamically stable at a rate of 40–60 beats per minute, such that temporary cardiac pacing may not be required. However, complete heart block following acute anterior myocardial infarction is more serious, and is associated with a high mortality (75%). Blockade in these cases usually results from infarction of the bundle branches, and escape rhythms originate low down in the ventricles. As such, they are slow (less than 45 beats/minute), irregular and the onset often occurs without warning. Temporary cardiac pacing is always required.

Atrio-ventricular Dissociation (Figure 4.10)

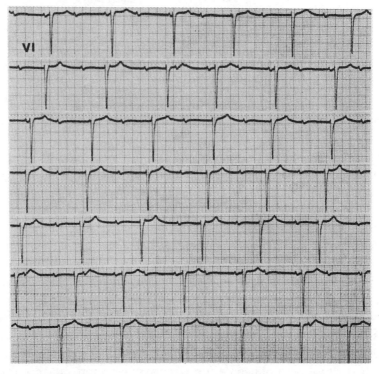

Figure 4.10 AV dissociation. Ventricular rate faster than atrial rate. P wave 'marches through' the QRS complex.

Rate: P wavw
Rate: Usually normal
Rhythm: Mostly regular
P Waves: Regular, unrelated to and slower than the *QRS* complex rate
PR Interval: Progressively shortens
QRS Complex: Normal morphology and at a faster rate than atria

Remarks: Atrio-ventricular dissociation (AVD) is a non-specific term used when the atria and ventricles are activated by independent pacemakers, the ventricular rate being the same or slightly faster than the atrial rate. In most cases, retrograde block prevents conduction of the ventricular impulse into the atria.

The rhythm is mostly regular, and manifests as normal *P* waves which bear no relation to the *QRS* complexes. As the sinus rate is slower than the ventricular rate, the *P–P* interval is longer than the *R–R* interval, and the *P* waves gradually overtake the *QRS* complexes. The *PR* interval diminishes, until the *P* wave become superimposed upon the *QRS* complex, and eventually appears on the other side (ie. the *P* wave marches through the *QRS* complex). Hence, AVD should always be expected when the *PR* interval progressively shortens.

When the *P* wave is far enough beyond the *QRS* complex, the sinus beat will 'capture' the next *QRS* complex, resulting in an early *PQRST* complex (called a 'capture beat').

Occasionally, synchronous discharge of the atria and ventricles will result in the two impulses meeting and interfering with each others progress, to produce a widened 'fusion beat'.

Atrio-ventricular dissociation (AVD) is often confused with complete heart block, as both show independent atrial and ventricular activity. However, in AVD the ventricular rate is faster than the atrial rate and there is no block at the AV junction, unless both the ventricular and atrial impulse stimulate the AV node at the same time, when it will become refractory. Long rhythm strips may be required to show this.

Demonstrating AVD is very important in the diagnosis of ventricular tachycardia (see Chapter 5).

Aetiology: AV dissociation may occur as an escape rhythm if there is slowing of the atrial impulses which allows emergence of a subsidiary pacemaker (eg. sino-atrial block). Alternatively it may result because of enhanced automaticity when there is acceleration of the rate of a subsidiary pacemaker (eg. as a result of myocardial ischaemia, or in response to drugs such as atropine or adrenaline).

Intra-ventricular Conduction Blocks

Disturbances of conduction are frequently found in patients with or without clinical evidence of heart disease. The term intra-ventricular conduction block refers to an impairment or complete block of conduction through one or more of the fascicles of the conducting tissue distal to the Bundle of His.

1. Bundle Branch Block

The main His bundle divides into two main bundle branches (left and right) which depolarize the ventricles, the left ventricle slightly before the right. Either of these bundles may become blocked resulting in asynchronous ventricular depolarization and contraction. As a consequence, the morphology of the *QRS* complex will alter to produce an 'M' or 'W' pattern over the blocked ventricle. The duration of the *QRS* complex will lengthen to more than 0.12 seconds and the *ST* segment is depressed and the *T* wave inverted over the blocked ventricle.

a) Left bundle branch block (LBBB)

When the left bundle branch is blocked, septal depolarization commences from right to left, instead of left to right as occurs normally. Hence, the initial *Q* wave in the left ventricular leads is lost and is replaced by a small upright *R* wave. The right ventricle is depolarized before the left (in contrast to normal), which produces an initial *R* wave in chest lead V1 and an *S* wave in lead V6. The left ventricle then depolarizes, producing an *S* wave in V1 and a second *R* wave (*R'*) in V6. The delay in bi-ventricular activation prolongs the *QRS* duration to > 0.12 seconds and alters the *QRS* morphology such that a 'W' shaped complex appears in V1 and an 'M' shaped complex in V6 (Figure 4.11). The *ST* segment is depressed and the *T* wave is inverted in leads V5 and V6 which overlie the left ventricle.

b) Right bundle branch block (RBBB)

If there is right bundle branch block, right ventricular depolarization is delayed, and occurs well after left ventricular depolarization. This late depolarization produces a secondary *R* wave (*R'*) in the right chest leads and a deep *S* wave in the left chest leads. The *QRS* is again prolonged to greater than 0.12 seconds, and the morphology

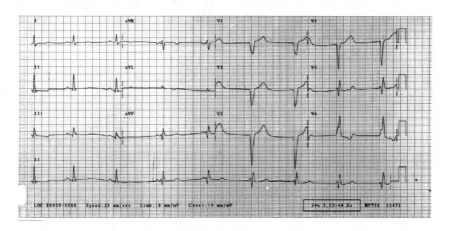

Figure 4.11 Left bundle branch block

is reversed such that in V1 it is an 'M' shaped complex, and in V6 it is a 'W' shaped complex (Figure 4.12). The *ST* segment is depressed and the *T* wave is inverted in the right ventricular leads.

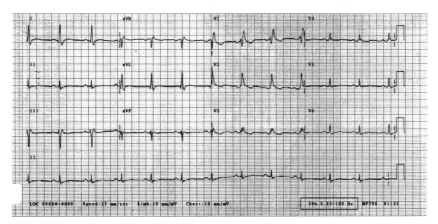

Figure 4.12 Right bundle branch block

2. Hemi-blocks

The left bundle divides into two hemi-fascicles, an anterior one running superio-laterally, and a posterior one running infero-medially. Each of these may become blocked, either on its own or in addition to the right bundle and left main bundles.

Although hemi-block leads to a slight prolongation of the *QRS* duration, this is usually not appreciated because the *QRS* duration is still less than 0.12 seconds. Recognition is therefore by a change in the frontal *QRS* axis which cannot be explained by any other cause.

The more common left anterior hemi-block is evident by left axis deviation to less than −30 degrees, whilst left posterior hemi-block produces right axis deviation in excess of +110 degrees. Additionally, *QRS* morphology may alter to show an *RS* pattern in lead I, and a *QR* in lead III if there is left posterior hemi-block, whilst in left anterior hemi-block an *RS* pattern is seen in standard lead III, and lead I has a *QR* complex.

3. Incomplete Bundle Branch Block

This term is commonly used when the morphology of the *QRS* complex is similar to that observed in established bundle branch block, but the *QRS* duration is within normal limits (< 0.12 seconds). The changes are not thought to be due to actual conduction block, but more indicative of delays produced in the depolarization of enlarged ventricles (eg. left ventricular hypertrophy).

Ventricular Standstill and Asystole

Rate: There is no ventricular rate
Rhythm: There is no ventricular rhythm
P Waves: Normal and regular (ventricular standstill), or absent (asystole)
PR Interval: None
QRS Complex: None

Remarks: If supra-ventricular impulses fail to reach the ventricles, ventricular standstill results unless a ventricular pacemaker takes over. Atrial *P* waves may continue to occur, but there will be no ventricular activity (Figure 4.13). This situation is sometimes referred to as tri-fascicular block.

More often, no activity either atrial or ventricular is seen, and the term asystole is then used (Figure 4.14). There is no cardiac output and cardiac arrest ensues.

About 25% of in-hospital and 10% of out-of-hospital cardiac arrests are due to asystole. It complicates up to 14% of cases of acute

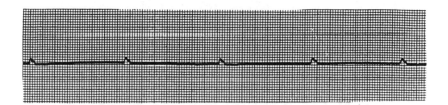

Figure 4.13 Ventricular standstill (tri-fascicular block)

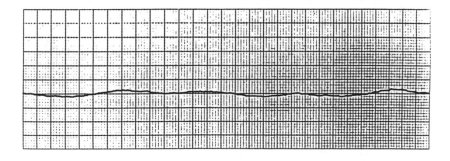

Figure 4.14 Asystole

myocardial infarction admitted to coronary care units, and the prognosis is very poor (mortality > 90%).

Aetiology: Myocardial ischaemia, metabolic acidosis, electrolyte imbalance, hypoxia, drugs.

A rhythm called *dying heart rhythm* (Figure 4.15) is sometimes seen terminally. True stimulation of the heart does not occur, and irregular, bizarre complexes continue to be seen on the ECG monitor for several minutes even though the patient is dead. For this reason, it may be better to turn the monitor off if relatives are present.

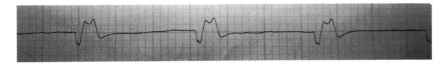

Figure 4.15 Dying heart rhythm

Chapter 5
Fast Heart
Rhythms

An increase in pulse rate (tachycardia) is the normal response of the heart to increased physical work so that the cardiac output may be increased. However, abnormal tachycardias are often associated with a diminished cardiac output. This is because at different heart rates, the proportion of the cardiac cycle occupied by systole remains remarkably constant, so that increases in heart rate occur at the expense of diastolic timing. Since ventricular filling takes place in diastole, as the heart rate increases the amount of time for ventricular filling falls and hence cardiac output is diminished. Furthermore, since coronary blood flow takes place during diastole, coronary insufficiency may result leading to ischaemic chest pain.

Symptoms provoked by tachycardia are determined less by the origin of the dysrhythmia and more by the heart rate and presence of underlying cardiac disease. Whilst many tachycardias may be asymptomatic, provoked symptoms may include angina, dyspnoea, palpitations or syncope. Myocardial ischaemia, heart failure and death are the major complications, whilst thrombo-embolism may be a risk in patients with atrial fibrillation, ventricular aneurysms or with tachycardias following acute myocardial infarction.

Mechanisms of Tachycardias

Most tachycardias are produced by one of two patho-physiological mechanisms, re-entry or enhanced automaticity.

a. Re-entry

Re-entry describes the circular movement of an impulse within the atria, within the ventricles, within AV junctional tissue or via an accessory pathway. This circus movement requires two or more conduction pathways with different electrical characteristics which permits the establishment of the re-entry circuit. Typically, there are two separate connections between the atria and the ventricles which allow forward (antegrade) conduction and return (retrograde) conduction. This is best understood by explaining the mechanism in relation to the Wolff-Parkinson-White syndrome. Here there is an anatomically separate AV conduction pathway called the Bundle of Kent which allows rapid AV transmission of the supra-ventricular impulse. The AV node allows normal transmission, but this is at a slower rate. The ventricles are therefore excited prematurely via the accessory pathway (pre-excitation). If a supraventricular ectopic beat occurs, it may find this accessory pathway refractory, and it will therefore be transmitted through the AV node, to depolarize the ventricles without pre-excitation. However, by the time this impulse has travelled slowly through the normal conducting tissue, the accessory pathway will have recovered, allowing the impulse to be conducted retrogradely into the atria. The atria will depolarize, and the generated impulse will re-enter the AV node, and a complete circuit will be set up, with rapid circus transmission initiating a tachycardia. Forward conduction takes place through the AV node and retrograde conduction through the accessory pathway (Figure 5.1).

Such a large re-entry circuit is very uncommon; Wolff-Parkinson-White syndrome affects 0.12% of the population. Most re-entry tachycardias are permitted by the establishment of a micro-circuit within or around the AV node itself (AV nodal re-entry tachycardias), which consist of only a few myocardial cells which allow circular conduction. Whilst these are not anatomically separate, electrically they provide the two pathways required for the re-entry circuit when part of the node becomes refractory. The rapid passage of the circulating impulse between the atria and ventricles results in what is sometimes called a reciprocating or re-entry tachycardia.

b. Enhanced Automaticity

Automaticity describes the inherent ability of specialised cardiac tissue to initiate electrical impulses by spontaneous depolarization. The responsible cells are known as pacemaker or automatic cells. In the sino-atrial node, these will discharge at about 80 times per minute, but elsewhere automatic cells have a slower spontaneous discharge rate. For example, in the AV node this may be at about 60 times per minute and within the ventricles about 30 times per minute. This back-up system of 'escape rhythms' exists to prevent rhythm

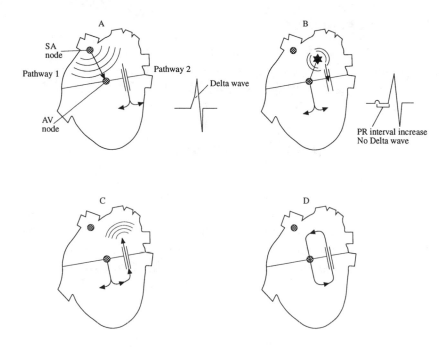

Figure 5.1 Diagram to show the mechanism of re-entry

Pathway 1 is the normal conduction pathway. The AV node is capable of conducting an impulse but with delay.

Pathway 2 is the accessory pathway (Bundle of Kent), which conducts atrial impulses to the ventricles without delay.

A) During sinus rhythm the impulse travels to the ventricles via the fast conducting accessory pathway. Pre-excitation is demonstrated on the resting ECG by a short PR interval and a delta wave.

B) A premature atrial ectopic occurs, and fails to be conducted through the accessory pathway because it is still refractory. It is therefore conducted normally to the ventricles via the slowly conducting AV node. The delay is often shown by a prolonged PR interval associated with the premature beat, followed by a normal QRS complex.

C) The premature impulse is now able to return retrogradely in the fast path way which is no longer refractory, and the atria are stimulated again.

D) The atrial impulse is then re-conducted to the ventricles through the AV node.

failure should the sino-atrial node fail to discharge. In this instance, an alternative pacemaker usually takes over, and although the rate will initially be slow, there is a tendency for the rate of this abnormal pacemaker to speed up because of 'enhanced automaticity'.

The Tachycardias

Electrocardiographically, the tachycardias may appear as narrow *QRS* complex tachycardias (*QRS* duration less than 0.12 seconds), or broad complex tachycardias (*QRS* duration longer than 0.12 seconds).

Narrow Complex Tachycardias

The main narrow complex tachycardias are junctional tachycardias, atrial flutter and atrial fibrillation. Each may present as a sustained or paroxysmal tachycardia. Treatment is usually directed towards the restoration of sinus rhythm, although in chronic or unstable rhythms, treatment aims to control the ventricular rate. Other causes of fast or irregular pulses include sinus tachycardia and multiple ectopic beats.

1. Sinus Tachycardia

Rate: 100–150 beats per minute
Rhythm: Regular
P Waves: Normal. At very fast rates the *P* waves may merge with the preceding *T* wave
PR Interval: Normal
QRS Complex: Normal

Remarks: Sinus tachycardia is arbitrarily defined as a sinus rhythm greater than 100 beats/minute, and commonly ranges between 100–150 beats/minute. A sinus tachycardia during exercise is of course normal, and young individuals can sometimes attain a rate in excess of 160 beats/minute. The maximal heart rate which a given individual may attain during peak exertion may be approximated by taking the patient's age from 220.

The *P* waves are normal and have a 1:1 relationship with the *QRS* complexes (Figure 5.2). The *PR* and *QT* intervals decrease as the

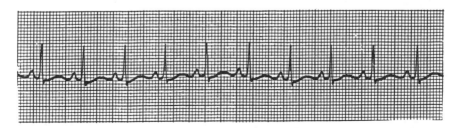

Figure 5.2 Sinus tachycardia

heart rate increases such that at very fast rates the *P* wave tends to merge with the preceding *T* wave. It may then be difficult to ascertain whether the rhythm is arising from the sinus node or an ectopic supra-ventricular focus, but there may be clues. During sinus tachycardia:

a)   The heart rate is usually less than 140 beats per minute and varies with respiration (sinus arrhythmia).

b)   The tachycardia is slow in onset and does not finish abruptly.

c)   The *P* waves are normal, and it may be possible to separate them from the *T* waves if pulse slowing exercises such as carotid sinus massage or the Valsalva manoeuvre are employed.

d)   *T* wave changes do not occur after cessation of the tachycardia. Abnormal tachycardias may leave *T* wave changes which last for days or weeks.

Aetiology: A sinus tachycardia is normal during exercise. At rest, a sinus tachycardia may be due to fever, anxiety, drugs (eg. atropine, catecholamines), pregnancy, anaemia, shock, thyrotoxicosis, myocardial infarction or heart failure.

2. Atrial Ectopic Beats

Rate: Usually normal
Rhythm: Irregularity caused by compensatory pauses
P Waves: Premature with abnormal shape or completely inverted. May be buried in the preceding *T* wave.
PR Interval: Usually normal but may vary from short to long
QRS Complex: Usually normal. Blocked beats occur if the AV node is refractory and the following *QRS* complex is then absent

Remarks: Atrial ectopic beats are very common in both health and disease, and occur when an atrial focus discharges before the sino-atrial pacemaker. The patient may or may not be aware of the feeling of a skipped or extra beat, which can be confirmed by feeling the pulse. On the ECG, atrial ectopic beats are seen as a premature, often abnormally shaped *P* wave, usually followed by a normal *QRS* complex (Figure 5.3). The further the ectopic focus is from the sinus node, the greater the abnormality in shape of the *P* wave, and the shorter the *PR* interval.

Conduction of atrial impulses to the ventricles depends upon the recovery status of the AV node. If the atrial ectopic beat arises near

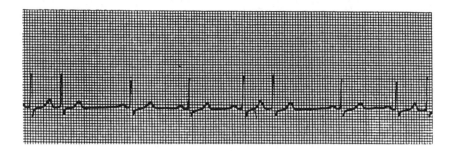

Figure 5.3 Atrial ectopic beats arising from two sites

the AV node (seen as an abnormal *P* wave and short PR interval) the AV node may be refractory. The impulse is therefore blocked and no *QRS* follows. If the AV node is partially refractory, a prolonged *PR* interval is seen because conduction of the ectopic beat is slowed. These atrial ectopics often precede sustained AV nodal tachycardias by initiation of a re-entry circuit.

Other parts of the conducting system below the AV node may also be refractory even when the AV node is able to convey the supra-ventricular impulse, and an aberrantly conducted impulse is then seen on the ECG.

Aberrant conduction is the term applied when a widened and abnormal *QRS* complex is seen following a supra-ventricular beat. It is the result of the unequal recovery periods of the right and left bundle branches. If a supra-ventricular stimulus is conducted to the bundles before both have recovered, bundle branch block will occur. This is usually of the right bundle branch block pattern since the right bundle has a longer refractory period than the left bundle. Differentiating ventricular ectopic beats from aberrantly conducted supra-ventricular beats may be difficult. With aberrantly conducted beats, *P* waves may be seen, and the *QRS* is usually of the right bundle branch block pattern. In chest lead V1, the R¹ wave is larger (ie. the right 'rabbit's ear' is longer). In contrast, ventricular ectopics usually show monophasic or bi-phasic *QRS* patterns in chest lead V1 and the left 'rabbit's ear' is longer (Figure 5.4). *P* waves are not seen and the ectopic beat is followed by a full compensatory pause.

Aetiology: Anxiety, stress, hypoxia, drugs (including smoking, alcohol, caffeine) and ischaemic heart disease.

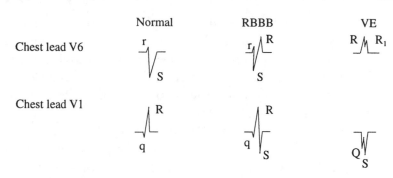

Figure 5.4 Normal V1 QRS patterns compared to right bundle branch block (RBBB) ventricular ectopics (VE)

3. Junctional (AV Nodal) Tachycardias

Sometimes it is not possible to determine the exact atrial rhythm during tachycardias unless specialised leads are used. Whilst narrow complex tachycardias are commonly labelled 'SVT's' (supra-ventricular tachycardias), they incorporate both ventricular and atrial myocardium within the circuit (with the exception of a true atrial tachycardia), and junctional or AV nodal tachycardias are better terms. The dysrhythmia is characterised by the sudden onset of a tachycardia greater than 150 beats/minute. In some patients there may be no symptoms, but the tachycardia may precipitate ischaemic pain, dyspnoea or syncope.

There are three forms of junctional tachycardia:

a)   AV nodal re-entry tachycardia
b)   AV re-entry tachycardia
c)   Accelerated junctional tachycardia.

a) AV nodal re-entry tachycardia (AVNRT)
Rate: 160–250 beats per minute
Rhythm: Regular
P Waves: Usually buried in the *QRST* complex
PR Interval: Usually not measurable
QRS Complex: Normal or aberrant

Remarks: Most junctional tachycardias are due to AV nodal re-entry, and originate from a focus within or immediately adjacent to the AV node. The re-entry circuit usually comprises a slow forward limb, and fast retrograde limb, resulting in almost simultaneous atrial and ventricular activation so that the *P* wave is usually buried in the *QRS* complex. The ECG shows rapid normal *QRS* complexes at a rate of 160–220 beats per minute. If visible, the *P* wave is represented by a small positive wave at the end of the *QRS* complex giving it the appearance of right bundle branch block. The onset (if recorded) is usually associated with a premature atrial beat which conducts to the ventricles with a prolonged *PR* interval.

A less common variant of the AVNRT is caused by a fast antegrade limb and slow retrograde limb. Atrial depolarization is therefore late, and the *P* wave appears after the *QRS* complex and is inverted in the inferior leads. It is sometimes referred to as a long *RP* tachycardia since the *PR* interval is less than the *RP'* interval.

b) Atrioventricular re-entry tachycardia (AVRT)

Rate: 160–250 beats per minute
Rhythm: Regular
P Waves: Abnormal. Often lost in preceding *QRST* complex
PR Interval: Usually not measurable
QRS Complex: Normal or aberrant

Remarks: AVRT's are associated with the presence of an accessory AV connection or pathway, such as the bundle of Kent in the Wolff-Parkinson-White syndrome. The diagnosis is often made from the sinus rhythm ECG (short *PR* interval and delta wave). During the tachycardia, slow antegrade conduction occurs through the AV node, and returns more quickly through a retrograde extra-nodal accessory pathway. The delta wave therefore disappears during the tachycardia since the antegrade conduction does not go through the accessory pathway. Atrial and ventricular activation are separated in time, which results in the *P* wave occurring between the *QRS* complexes. Often the *P* waves are difficult to see, but brief interruptions of the tachycardia (for example by carotid sinus massage) may be very helpful.

c) Accelerated junctional (idio-nodal) tachycardia

Rate: A junctional escape rhythm has a rate of 40–60 beats per minute, which usually speeds up to 60–100 beats per minute (idio-nodal tachycardia)
Rhythm: Regular
P Waves: May be seen before, after or within the *QRS* complex
PR Interval: None or short
QRS Complex: Normal

Remarks: If there is suppression of sinus or atrial pacemaker function, the AV node may take over as the pacemaker. The normal discharge rate from the AV junction is about 50–60 beats per minute. The junctional impulse is conducted backwards to the atria and forwards to the ventricles. If the impulse depolarizes the atria first, the *P* wave is seen in front of the *QRS* complex. If the ventricles are depolarized first, the *P* wave occurs after the *QRS* complex. The *P* wave is hidden within the *QRS* complex if atria and ventricles are simultaneously discharged. Junctional escape is not a very dependable rhythm, and although often well tolerated may compromise cardiac output. Because of enhanced automaticity, the rate may increase gradually to 70–100 beats/minute (Figure 5.5). The sinus node often continues to discharge at a slower rate, and there is a propensity to AV dissociation with capture beats appearing. *QRS* complexes are usually normal, unless there is aberrant conduction.

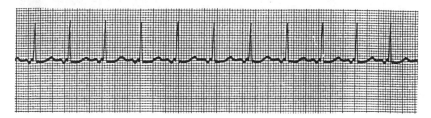

Figure 5.5 Junctional (nodal) tachycardia. Note the inverted P waves

Aetiology of junctional tachycardias: Most junctional tachycardias occur in normal hearts, with episodes often starting in early adult life and persisting randomly throughout life. There is an association with mitral valve prolapse.

Junctional escape arises as a consequence of sinus node depression (eg. drugs, ischaemia), and accelerated junctional rhythm is most often seen with digoxin toxicity, but can occur following cardiac surgery and myocardial infarction.

4. Paroxysmal Atrial Tachycardia (PAT)

Rate: Atrial rate is 150–250 beats per minute, but AV block may reduce the ventricular rate to under 100 beats per minute.
Rhythm: Regular
P Waves: Abnormal, and often lost in preceding *QRST* complex
PR Interval: Usually not measurable
QRS Complex: Normal or aberrant

Remarks: The term paroxysmal atrial tachycardia was often incorrectly applied to AVNRTs in the past. True paroxysmal atrial tachycardia is much less common, and is caused by the rapid discharge of an atrial pacemaker, usually in the inter-atrial septum (Figure 5.6). It is therefore a true supra-ventricular tachycardia.

An intra-atrial re-entry circuit is usually present, often initiated by frequent atrial ectopic beats. A few cases of atrial tachycardia may be caused by enhanced automaticity of an atrial focus which speeds up (usually in patients with digoxin toxicity). If second degree atrio-ventricular block is present, the ventricular response is usually not rapid and causes little systemic upset.

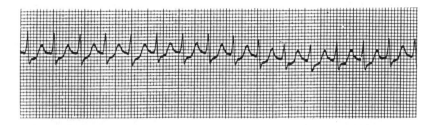

Figure 5.6 Atrial tachycardia

Aetiology: Paroxysmal atrial tachycardias at fast rates (1:1 conduction) often occur in young patients with no cardiac disease. The tachycardia may be caused by stress, anxiety states, drugs (including alcohol, tobacco) and fatigue. The tachycardia is usually well tolerated. In patients with cardiac disease, the AV node is usually unable to conduct all impulses, and atrial tachycardia with second degree AV block occurs. 'PAT with block' is a classic rhythm disturbance caused by digoxin toxicity.

5. Atrial Flutter

Rate: Ventricular rate varies according to AV conduction, typically 70–150 per minute
Rhythm: Regular unless AV conduction changes
P Waves: *F* (flutter) waves at 250–400 per minute; discrete *F* waves may be visible only in some leads (especially V1)
PR Interval: None, although the *FR* interval may vary in a Wenckebach-type pattern
QRS Complex: Normal or aberrant

Remarks: During atrial flutter, the atria usually contract at a rate of about 300/minute. The ECG shows flutter (*F*) waves which have a

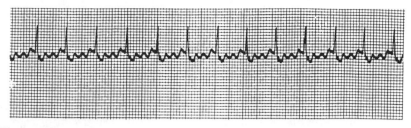

Figure 5.7 Atrial flutter

saw-tooth appearance in the inferior leads (Figure 5.7). Leads V1 and
V2 often appear to show large discrete bi-phasic *P* waves, suggesting
sinus tachycardia. In addition, flutter waves may be obscured by the
QRST complex and because atrial activity is concealed, sinus tachycardia of 150 beats/minute may be diagnosed. In such cases, flutter
waves may be revealed by carotid sinus massage, which will transiently increased AV blockade and slow the ventricular response
(Figure 5.8). If this is not effective, alternate *F* waves should be sought,
and are often found hidden in the preceding *T* wave. This may be
confirmed by measuring the interval between the *P* wave and the
following *T* wave peak. It should be precisely the same as the interval
between the *T* wave peak and the following *P* wave.

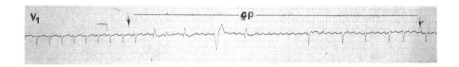

Figure 5.8 The effect of carotid sinus massage

Although the AV node can respond to atrial rates of about 300
beats/minute, there is usually some degree of AV blockade. In the
healthy AV node unaffected by drugs, this results in a ventricular rate
of about 150 beats/minute (ie. there is 2:1 block). Higher degrees of AV
blockade usually occur in the presence of drugs, or when there is
damage to the conducting system, although 3:1 conduction is unusual.
Whilst the pulse is usually regular, AV conduction ratios may vary,
giving rise to varying *R–R* intervals on the ECG and an irregular pulse.

Exercise decreases AV blockade and may lead to a doubling of
the pulse rate. As a result, the apparently normal patient with a pulse
rate of 75 beats per minute may feel faint on exercise when switching
from 4:1 block to 2:1 conduction. During 2:1 conduction, ventricu-

lar conduction may become aberrant and the widened *QRS* complexes may give the appearance of ventricular tachycardia.

Mural thrombi may form, since atrial contraction is not as strong as usual and stasis of blood occurs.

Aetiology: Usually associated with acute or chronic atrial dilatation as complicates cardio-respiratory disorders such as coronary heart disease, cardiomyopathy, cor pulmonale and pulmonary embolism.

6. Atrial Fibrillation

Rate: Ventricular rates vary from very slow to very fast depending on AV conduction
Rhythm: Irregularly irregular
P Waves: None – replaced by fibrillatory (f) waves
PR Interval: None
QRS: Normal but aberrant conduction is common at fast ventricular rates

Remarks: Paroxysmal or sustained atrial fibrillation is one of the most common cardiac dysrhythmias. It is more frequent with increasing age, affecting about 2% of people over 60 years of age.

During atrial fibrillation, normal atrial contraction is replaced by a disorganised and continuous series of irregular fibrillation waves (350–600 per minute), which is ineffective for atrial emptying and functionally the atria remain in diastole. The loss of atrial systole limits ventricular filling, and stretching prior to ventricular contraction, and hence the presence of atrial fibrillation may reduce the cardiac output by up to 20%.

Although atrial fibrillation makes the heart less efficient, the most important consequence is that of thrombo-embolism, especially stroke. Peripheral embolisation is particularly high in patients with paroxysmal atrial fibrillation, rheumatic heart disease and thyrotoxicosis.

The ECG in atrial fibrillation shows the replacement of *P* waves by small irregular undulations of the baseline (f waves) which repre-

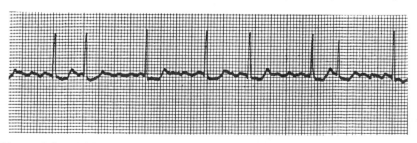

Figure 5.9 Atrial fibrillation

sent the only evidence of atrial activity (Figure 5.9). This is not always visible in all leads. Sometimes, the *f* waves are very coarse, and may be mistaken for normal *P* waves, or *F* (flutter) waves. If the atrial *f* waves have a rate of greater than 350/minute, atrial fibrillation is more likely, particularly if the ventricular response is totally irregular.

At fast heart rates, the ventricular response becomes more regular and *f* waves are usually not visible. Differentiation from a nodal tachycardia may then be difficult, and often it is only a slight irregularity in the ventricular rate which allows the correct diagnosis to be made. The only occasion when the ventricular rate will be regular is when atrial fibrillation is complicated by complete heart block.

The ventricular response in the untreated patient with atrial fibrillation is usually at a rate of about 100–180 beats/minute. The *QRS* is usually normal, but at fast ventricular rates, aberrant conduction often occurs.

Aetiology: Amongst the more frequent causes of atrial fibrillation are ischaemic heart disease, thyrotoxicosis, mitral valve disease, hypertensive heart disease and constrictive pericarditis. It may also be precipitated by an acute intra-thoracic process, such as a chest infection or pulmonary embolism. Lone atrial fibrillation is said to occur when there is no recognisable underlying cause.

Broad Complex Tachycardias

Broad complex tachycardias are normally of ventricular origin. Occasionally they may be produced when supraventricular tachycardias are aberrantly conducted to the ventricles, or occur in the presence of pre-existing bundle branch block.

Ventricular dysrhythmias are particularly common following acute myocardial infarction and are sometimes fatal. Their detection and prompt treatment was the primary reason for the creation of cardiac care units. Other factors which predispose patients to ventricular dysrhythmias include chronic myocardial ischaemia, electrolyte imbalance, acid–base abnormalities, hypoxia and certain drugs.

a) Myocardial ischaemia and injury

Myocardial ischaemia may result from occlusive or non-occlusive changes in the coronary vasculature (eg. coronary atheroma or coronary artery spasm) which impair the blood supply to the myocardium. Ischaemia predisposes to cardiac dysrhythmias regardless of whether or not necrosis takes place. Normal electrical conduction pathways may alter with ischaemia and provide a focus for dysrhythmias. Hypoxia, hypo-glycaemia, cold and other physiological stresses may exert a reflex catecholamine release which makes ectopic activity more common. Myocardial irritability following acute myocardial infarction is, of course, a major cause of ventricular dysrhythmias. Necrotic myocardial tissue provides a focus for this ectopic activity, and myocardial hypoxia associated with exaggerated catecholamine release compounds the situation.

b) Electrolyte and acid–base imbalance

i) Calcium imbalance

Hypo-calcaemia reduces myocardial contractility and abnormal tachycardias are common. It prolongs ventricular systole which recognised on the ECG by prolongation of the *QT* interval. The *T* wave may become inverted. Widening of the *QRS* complex occurs with severe hypo-calcaemia.

Hyper-calcaemia on the other hand is associated with bradycardias, including heart block and asystole. Hypercalcaemia causes ventricular systole to shorten (ie. the *QT* interval shortens), and the *T* wave becomes wide and inverted. Hyper-calcaemia potentiates digoxin toxicity.

ii) Potassium imbalance

The earliest ECG sign of increasing hyper-kalaemia is a progressive increase in height of the *T* wave which becomes peaked or tented. The *R* wave diminishes in size, the *S* wave becomes deeper and the *QT* interval shortens. Finally, the *P* wave flattens and eventually disappears. The *QRS* widens indicating an intra-ventricular conduction block. If untreated, the *QRS* duration continues to increase and ventricular fibrillation ensues.

A low serum potassium concentration is probably the most common electrolyte disturbance seen in hospital practice. With progressive hypo-kalaemia, the *QT* interval lengthens and the *ST* segment becomes depressed and trough-like. The *T* wave flattens and the *U* wave becomes prominent.

Untreated hypo-kalaemia can lead to ventricular ectopic beats, atrial tachycardia and eventually ventricular tachycardia and fibrillation.

iii) Acid–base imbalance

The acid–base status may be affected by changes in respiration or metabolism. Hypoxia and electrolyte imbalance make dysrhythmias more likely. For example, acidosis increases calcium ionisation and causes hyper-kalaemia. In addition, acidaemia reduces the effect of catecholamines on the heart (ie. it is negatively inotropic).

c) The effect of drugs

Many drugs, both cardiovascular and non-cardiovascular, may predispose the patient to cardiac dysrhythmias. Further, many drugs prescribed as anti-dysrhythmic agents may sometimes produce serious dysrhythmias (pro-arrhythmic effect).

The most frequent drug effect seen in the ECG is with digoxin therapy. The *QT* interval shortens, the *ST* segment sags, and the *T* wave merges with the *ST* segment. The *PR* also becomes prolonged. Beta-blockers, quinidine and procainamide may prolong the *QT* interval and flatten the *T* wave. Ventricular tachycardia may be precipitated by drugs which affect the *QT* interval, such as Class 1 anti-dysrhythmic agents (disopyramide, quinidine), phenothiazines, as well as low levels of calcium, potassium and magnesium. It is likely that it is severe left ventricular dysfunction which predisposes to these episodes of non-sustained ventricular tachycardia which may sometimes progress to ventricular fibrillation.

1. Ventricular Ectopics

Rate: Normal

Rhythm: Irregularity caused by ectopics followed by compensatory pause

P Waves: Do not precede ectopic beats, but may be produced by retrograde conduction of the ventricular beat into the atria and then seen as an inverted *P* wave

PR Interval: None

QRS Complex: Widened and abnormally shaped. *T* wave in opposite direction

Remarks: Ventricular extra-systoles occur when an ectopic ventricular focus discharges prematurely anywhere within the His-Purkinje system or the ventricles. They can occur at any time in diastole. The *QRS* complex is premature, widened (> 0.12 seconds), slurred and usually notched. There is no preceding *P* wave, and the following *T* wave usually points in the opposite direction (Figure 5.10). The morphology of each ventricular ectopic is usually identical if the focus is solitary. Ectopics of differing morphology usually arise from multiple ventricular sites (multi-focal ectopics), although ectopics

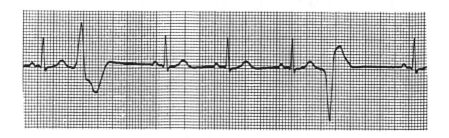

Figure 5.10 Ventricular ectopic beats arising from two sites

from the same area may have different shapes because of being conducted in a different pattern, and the term 'multi-form ectopics' is probably better than multi-focal ectopics.

Ventricular ectopic beats are followed by a full compensatory pause since the sino-atrial node is not penetrated by retrograde activity. The next sinus beat occurs at the expected time, and the *R–R* interval between the preceding and following complexes is twice the normal *R–R* interval.

Ventricular bigeminy consists of paired beats one sinus and one a ventricular ectopic. When separated by two or three normal beats, the terms trigeminy and quadrigeminy are used.

Coupling intervals

The coupling interval refers to the time interval between each ventricular ectopic and non-ectopic beat. Ventricular ectopics arising from a single focus are usually identical in shape and have a fixed coupling interval (variation < 0.08 seconds). These ectopic beats do not seem to precede ventricular fibrillation. However, couplets and salvoes of ventricular ectopic beats (pairs or multiples) which have differing morphologies and do not demonstrate fixed coupling intervals may predispose to ventricular tachycardia and fibrillation.

The R-on-T phenomenon

The *R-on-T* phenomenon refers to a ventricular ectopic occurring on the apex of the preceding *T* wave, a vulnerable period which sometimes results in ventricular fibrillation.

Complex ventricular ectopics

If ventricular ectopic beats are multiform, *R-on-T* or occurring in salvoes, they are described as complex. Unifocal ventricular ectopic beats frequently occur in healthy individuals, and may be considered normal. However, complex ventricular ectopics more usually associated with cardiac disease.

Aetiology: Routine prolonged ECG monitoring of apparently healthy individuals will reveal ventricular ectopic beats in more than half, and 10% of these will be multi-form. Non-cardiac causes include febrile illnesses, excessive consumption of tea, coffee, alcohol and cigarettes, and precipitated by drugs including tri-cyclic anti-depressants, digoxin and broncho-dilators (salbutamol, aminophyline, etc.). Ventricular ectopics may associate with cardiac disorders such as myocardial ischaemia, aortic valve disease and mitral valve prolapse.

2. Parasystole

Rate: Normal
Rhythm: Mostly regular
P Waves: Regular and dissociated
PR Interval: Not measurable
QRS Complex: Widened

Remarks: Parasystole is a dual rhythm where two pacemakers concurrently and independently govern the rhythm of the heart. It is usually an automatic ectopic ventricular focus which discharges regularly and competes with a second focus which is located in the atria, the AV junction or the ventricles. Usually competition is with normal sinus rhythm, the ventricular rhythm usually being at a slightly faster rate. The interval between successive ventricular ectopic beats is the same or a multiple of that interval, and since this parasystolic focus is independent of the regular heart rhythm, there is no fixed relationship between the two rhythms and the coupling interval varies (ie. the interval between the ectopic beat and the sinus beat).

It might be expected that the dominant pacemaker would take over cardiac rhythm and suppress the ectopic focus. However, during parasystole, the ectopic focus is protected by 'entrance block', a uni-directional block in the vicinity of the ectopic focus. Outward conduction from the ectopic focus is normal and forms the secondary pacemaker. Two pacemakers therefore exist, each discharging at their own independent rate and depolarizing the myocardium if it is in a responsive state. If the two pacemakers discharge simultaneously, each activates the adjacent myocardium, and a 'fusion beat' will arise as the two discharge wave-fronts collide. A *QRS* complex intermediate in appearance between a normal sinus beat and a ventricular ectopic results (Figure 5.11).

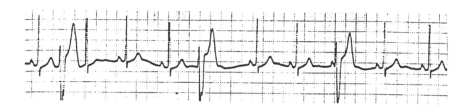

Figure 5.11 Parasystole (showing fusion beats and capture beats)

Aetiology: Parasystole is relatively uncommon, but may be seen following myocardial infarction and in patients taking digoxin.

3. Ventricular Tachycardia

Rate: 140–250 per minute
Rhythm: Regular (should not vary by more than 0.04 seconds)
P Waves: AV dissociation, with regular unrelated *P* waves sometimes being seen
PR Interval: None
QRS Complex: Widened and abnormal

Remarks: Ventricular tachycardia is a serious re-entry dysrhythmia which may be defined as a succession of five or more beats arising from one or more foci in the ventricles at a rate of over 120 beats/minute. The *QRS* complexes are wide (> 0.12 seconds) and regular at a rate of 140–250 beats/minute. A *monomorphic* ventricular tachycardia has uniform beat to beat morphology, whereas a *polymorphic* ventricular tachycardia has a constantly changing, sometimes subtle beat-to-beat *QRS* configuration.

During ventricular tachycardia, the atria continue to beat and dissociated *P* waves may be seen. The atrial rate is usually slower than the ventricular rate, originating at the sinus node. However, there may be co-existent atrial tachycardia, junctional rhythm or atrial fibrillation. Occasionally, ventricular beats may pass back through the AV node to stimulate the atria and *P* waves then appear after the *QRS* complex.

Fusion and capture beats may be present, which helps considerably in distinguishing ventricular tachycardia from other broad complex tachycardias.

Fusion beats occur when a normal supra-ventricular stimulus collides with a ventricular stimulus being conducted retrogradely. The resulting *QRS* complex looks partly like a normal *QRS* complex and partly like a ventricular ectopic beat.

Capture beats occur when an atrial stimulus arrives at a non-refractory AV node and is conducted normally to the ventricles. This results in a normal *P* wave followed by a normal (narrow) *QRS* complex.

The tachycardia may be sustained or non-sustained. *Sustained ventricular tachycardias* persist for over 30 seconds and lead to haemodynamic collapse, whereas a *non-sustained ventricular tachycardia* spontaneously terminates within 30 seconds and is not associated with significant haemodynamic disturbance.

There are four types of ventricular tachycardia (VT):

a)   Monomorphic ventricular tachycardia
b)   Polymorphic ventricular tachycardia
c)   Accelerated idio-ventricular tachycardia (slow VT)
d)   Ventricular flutter.

a) Monomorphic (extra-systolic) ventricular tachycardia

This is the most common form of ventricular tachycardia. Each paroxysm of VT starts with a ventricular ectopic beat which occurs at the same fixed interval from the previous *QRS* complex. The complexes are of uniform appearance (monomorphous), and each episode of VT continues for a variable time, usually terminating with a long pause before sinus rhythm returns (Figure 5.12).

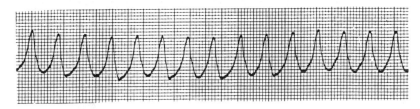

Figure 5.12 Monomorphic ventricular tachycardia

b) Polymorphic ventricular tachycardia (torsade de pointes)

Torsade de pointes ('turning of the points') is characterised by paroxysms of ventricular tachycardia following a *QRST* complex with a prolonged *QT* interval (Figure 5.13). The episodes may be precipitated by drugs which prolong the *QT* interval such as Class 1 antidysrhythmic agents (quinidine, procainamide, disopyramide), phenothiazines or electrolyte imbalance. A congenital prolongation of the *QT* interval may occasionally be the cause (Romano-Ward syndrome).

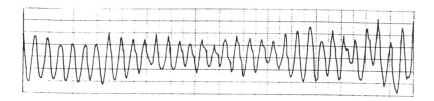

Figure 5.13 Torsade de pointes (polymorphic ventricular tachycardia). Note the changing amplitude of the complexes

The *QRS* complexes undulate around the iso-electric line with a marked change of amplitude occurring every 5–30 beats following *QRS* complexes demonstrating the prolonged *QT* interval. Torsade de pointes usually terminates spontaneously but may precede ventricular fibrillation.

Distinguishing torsade de pointes from other types of ventricular tachycardia is important, since usual drug therapy often makes the situation worse.

c) Accelerated idio-ventricular tachycardia

If there is failure of impulse formation from higher pacemaker centres, the ventricles take over with a slow, unreliable pacemaker at 30–40 beats per minute (Figure 5.14). This may last for a few seconds, or may be continuous with a predisposition to asystole.

An accelerated idio-ventricular rhythm is induced by enhanced automaticity which is faster than the inherent ventricular rate. The rate does not usually exceed 120 beats/minute, and is often referred to as slow ventricular tachycardia (Figure 5.15). After about 30 beats sinus rhythm usually takes over, although it may be replaced by sustained ventricular tachycardia or ventricular fibrillation.

d) Ventricular flutter

Ventricular flutter is characterised by a rapid ventricular rate of

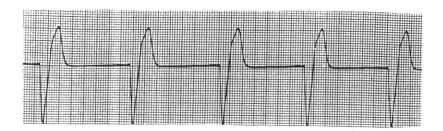

Figure 5.14 Idio-ventricular rhythm

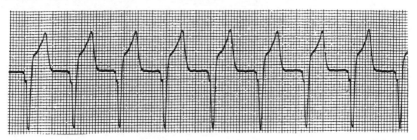

Figure 5.15 Accelerated idio-ventricular rhythm (slow ventricular tachycardia)

180–250 beats per minute, where it is not possible to differentiate the *QRS* complexes from the *ST* segments or *T* waves. The pattern of oscillating waves of large amplitude has been likened to rows of hair pins (Figure 5.16). It often precedes ventricular fibrillation.

Aetiology of ventricular tachycardia: Usually coronary artery disease. Accelerated idio-ventricular tachycardias often follow inferior myocardial infarction, and may be a feature of coronary reperfusion following successful thrombolysis. It is rarely seen otherwise.

Other causes of ventricular tachycardia include myocarditis, cardiomyopathy, mitral valve disease, intra-cardiac instrumentation, drugs (eg. digoxin, sympathomimetic amines and phenothiazines). Metabolic causes (electrolyte imbalance, hypoxia, acidaemia) should also be considered.

Benign ventricular tachycardia is said to occur when there is a normal resting ECG, a normal *QT* interval, no evidence of structural heart disease and no significant haemodynamic symptoms.

Correctly Diagnosing Broad Complex Tachycardias

Differentiating ventricular tachycardia from other broad complex tachycardias is important both in the management of the acute dysrhythmia and for long-term therapy to prevent recurrence.

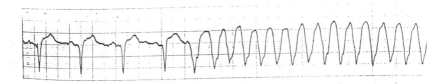

Figure 5.16 Ventricular flutter (rate 220). This episode has been precipitated by a ventricular eptopic falling on the end of sinus beat (R-on-P phenomenon)

Regular broad complex tachycardias may be due to:

a)   Ventricular tachycardia
b)   SVT with pre-existent bundle branch block
c)   SVT with rate related bundle branch block.

Irregular broad-complex tachycardias may be due to:

a)   atrial fibrillation with pre-existing bundle branch block
b)   atrial fibrillation with rate related bundle branch block
c)   torsade de pointes.

Ventricular tachycardia is often misdiagnosed as having a supra-ventricular origin, which is of major concern since treatment and prognosis are markedly different. Generally speaking, if the patient is known to have cardiac disease, then it is wise to assume that the broad complex tachycardias is ventricular tachycardia. If the patient is thought to have a normal heart, the tachycardia is more likely to be supra-ventricular in origin.

Differentiation relies heavily on the demonstration of independent atrial and ventricular activity (AV dissociation).

A full 12-lead ECG should always be recorded provided the patient is well enough during the tachycardia. If the *QRS* in sinus rhythm was of normal duration, a *QRS* duration > 0.14 seconds during the tachycardia indicates a ventricular origin. Ventricular concordance (uniformly positive or negative *QRS* complexes) in the chest leads is virtually diagnostic of ventricular tachycardia. The

Table 5.1 Features of Ventricular Tachycardia

A) Clinically
  The venous pulse rate is slower than the arterial pulse rate
  There are irregular cannon waves seen in the venous pulse
  There is varying intensity of the first heart sound

B) In the 12 lead ECG
  There is left axis deviation (*QRS* < −30 degrees)
  The *QRS* duration is > 0.14 seconds (140 milliseconds)
  There are multiple *QRS* morphologies
  There is concordance of the *QRS* vector in the chest leads (ie.they are all in the same direction)
  In chest lead V1, the *R* wave is taller than the *R^l* wave (the left 'rabbit's ear' is longer)
  Dissociated *P* waves may be seen (AV dissociation)
  Blocked, fusion and capture beats may be present
  There is a *Q* wave in V6 or a notch on the downstroke of the *S* wave in V1/V2

R–R interval is regular unless there are capture beats, and in contrast to supra-ventricular tachycardias (which are affected by respiration) does not vary by more than 0.04 seconds.

It is important to realise that the clinical condition of the patient is not helpful. Some patients tolerate ventricular tachycardia extremely well, whilst others may be severely haemodynamically compromised by a rapid supra-ventricular tachycardia.

If in doubt, broad complex tachycardias should be treated as ventricular tachycardia.

Guidelines for diagnosis are shown in Table 5.1.

4. Ventricular Fibrillation

Rate: None
Rhythm: None
P Waves: None
QRS Complex: None

Remarks: Ventricular fibrillation (VF) is the most serious dysrhythmia, since death results if it is not terminated rapidly. Electrically and mechanically, the heart is completely disorganised when in ventricular fibrillation and cardiac arrest results. The ECG shows fine or coarse waves of irregular size, shape and rhythm (Figure 5.17). Fine VF may mimic asystole and produce an apparent flat line on the ECG monitor.

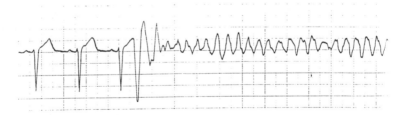

Figure 5.17 Ventricular fibrillation

*Aetiology:*Ventricular fibrillation is the most common cause of out-of-hospital cardiac arrest (75%), and although many have evidence of coronary heart disease, less than half seem to have had an acute myocardial infarction. In contrast, about 90% of deaths following acute myocardial infarction are due to ventricular fibrillation, nearly half of which occur in the first hour following onset of symptoms and most immediately (acute occlusional ventricular fibrillation).

Primary ventricular fibrillation describes fibrillation which occurs within the first 12 hours of acute myocardial infarction. It is usually associated with a good prognosis if reversed rapidly, as the heart is often still functioning well.

Re-perfusional ventricular fibrillation may occur following thrombolysis, but paradoxically this probably reflects a good prognosis; the infarct related artery has been opened.

Secondary or late ventricular fibrillation describes fibrillation in hearts whose function has been severely compromised by the infarct (ie. there is often heart failure or hypotension). The long-term prognosis is poor.

Other causes of ventricular fibrillation include those causing ventricular tachycardia, as well as drug overdoses, electrocution, hypoxia and acidaemia.

Chapter 6
Ambulatory Monitoring of Cardiac Rhythm

Ambulatory monitoring of cardiac rhythm is a technique by which cardiac rate, rhythm and *QRST* morphology can be evaluated whilst the patient is exercising and preferably during their normal daily activities. Static bedside monitors are obviously of limited value in detecting short or infrequent rhythm disturbances, especially if induced by exertion or stressful situations.

The major role of ambulatory ECG monitoring is in the evaluation of symptoms suggestive of a paroxysmal cardiac dysrhythmia. Most commonly, this is in the investigation of transient neurological symptoms which might be attributable to falls in cardiac output such as syncope and dizziness. Monitoring aims to establish a relationship between symptoms and accompanying disturbances in cardiac rhythm. Other cardiac symptoms often investigated by ambulatory electrocardiography include atypical chest pain, episodic shortness of breath and palpitations. The technique may also be utilised to assess the efficacy or pro-arrhythmic effects of anti-dysrhythmic drugs with tapes being performed before and after treatment.

Dynamic Electrocardiography: The Role of the Ambulatory Monitor

An American called Norman 'Jeff' Holter was the first to suggest the role of portable ECG recorders in the late 1940s, and hence these machines are often known as 'Holter monitors'. Other epithets include 24 hour tapes (referring to the normal recording period), ambulatory monitors or dynamic electrocardiograms, the latter two probably being preferred terms. From the initial bulky, short duration recorders, these monitors have been refined to light, small strong machines capable of recording the heart rhythm continuously for prolonged periods. The tape recorder is not very obtrusive Figure 6.1 and is easily carried in a harness.

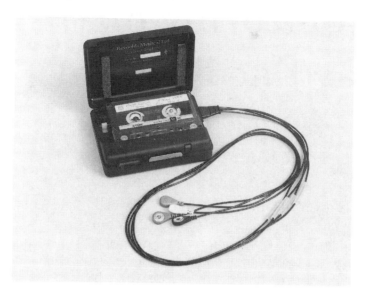

Figure 6.1 Holter monitor (Reproduced by kind permission of Reynolds Medical Ltd)

The Electrode System

A bipolar electrode system is utilised employing three, four or five skin sensors depending upon whether one or two-channel ECG recording is being carried out, the latter being more usual. The two exploring electrodes are placed to record a modified V1 and V5 chest lead, with the two indifferent electrodes being placed over the manubrium and the right side of the chest (Figure 6.1a). The modified V1 lead will produce excellent P wave morphology and the second channel (V5) allows QRS axis changes to be detected if there is an intra-ventricular conduction defect or if there are episodes of ventricular pre-excitation.

Excellent reproduction of the ST segment has been difficult in the past, but now this has been much improved so that monitoring ST segment shift is another important indication for use of these monitors. Abnormal ST segment displacement has been found to be relatively specific for myocardial ischaemia, occurring in less than 5% of healthy individuals. ST segment monitoring is used to document

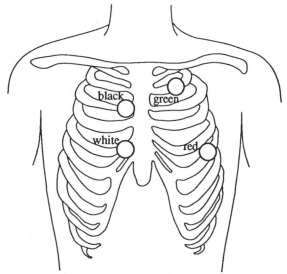

Suitable for arrhythmia and ST analysis

Modified V5   Modified V1

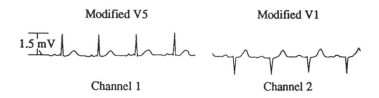

Channel 1   Channel 2

Adjust if necessary to obtain ideal ECG for analysis

Figure 6.1a Electrode placement during Holter monitoring

symptomatic and silent myocardial ischaemia; as many as two-thirds of ischaemia episodes have been found to be asymptomatic.

Method of Recording

An ordinary tape cassette and new batteries are inserted into the machine and the monitor is tested. It is often of value to make initial recordings with the patient sitting, standing and lying, since QRS morphology may vary substantially with body position. Recording these first will produce a baseline when the whole tape is later analysed. The patient is instructed to carry on normal daily activities. A detailed diary for the day's activities is usually kept (eg. sleeping, working, watching television) with clear descriptions and timing of any symptoms, especially faintness, palpitations and breathlessness. Some machines have 'event markers', a button which may be pressed by the patient to mark the tape at the onset of symptoms so that the cardiac rhythm at that exact time is documented. The diary of timed symptoms and the referral note are of major value during tape analysis and interpretation.

The typical 24 hour recording provides about 100,000 complexes for analysis, but fortunately high speed computerised electro-cardioscanners are available to aid tape analysis (Figure 6.2). These machines work in different ways, but the most common uses a system called 'AVSEP' (audio-visual superimposed electrocardio-graphic presentation) which superimposes successive *PQRS* cycles on an oscilloscope screen. The computer detects the normal *QRS* which is stored in the memory, and then other *QRS* complexes are compared with the original. Similarly, the *R–R* interval is logged and compared with other *R–R* intervals. When the morphology of the *QRS* complex differs, the visual signal of the abnormality interrupts the otherwise uniform pattern which is readily seen. In addition, an audio signal can be made to sound with each detected complex and any change in *QRS* frequency alters the pitch of the note. The recording may then be stopped and a rhythm strip obtained. Other scanners may use groups of *QRS* complexes or may be able to auto-matically sample at pre-selected intervals and wherever an 'event marker' is found. Most machines now have computerised automatic dysrhythmia recognition units which are able to carry out ectopic counts and detailed rhythm analysis (Figure 6.3).

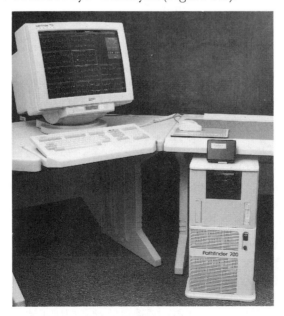

Figure 6.2 ECG interpretation unit (Reproduced by kind permission of Reynolds Medical Ltd)

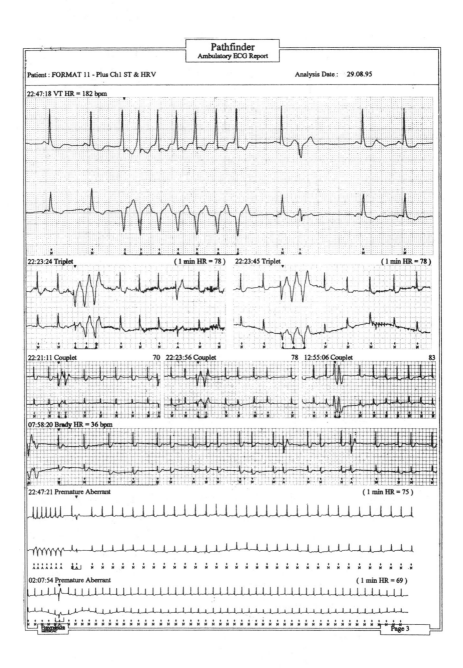

Figure 6.3 Print-out of tape

The analysers are usually overseen by a skilled operator during high speed tape replay when a 24 hour period may be viewed in under 10 minutes, although selection of rhythm strips and print out make full processing a little longer. Analysis may be fully automatic when the machine will print excerpts from the tape according to pre-set criteria, semi-automatic when the selection of events may be kept or rejected according to the technicians view of their importance, or interventional, when the technician may interrupt the tape when-ever a significant event takes place. Presentation of the contents may be made in many different ways. Sample normal rhythms and dysrhythmias are printed on standard ECG paper, with precise timing of symptoms to allow comparison with the patient's diary to correlate symptoms and dysrhythmias. A full disclosure record will display the whole 24 hour recording in miniature, which is some-times of value in picking out episodic dysrhythmias.

Other Recording Methods

Holter monitoring is limited both by recording capacity and by the fact that events must take place during the period of study. Patients frequently complain that 'It never happens when I'm attached to the recorder'. Fortunately several modified recording devices have been developed which aid dysrhythmia detection.

1) Event recorders

Event recorders are able to record for about 30 minutes total dura-tion, but instead of running continuously can be manually activated at the onset of symptoms or will activate automatically should any sudden change in rate or rhythm occur (according to pre-set crite-ria). In the past, these devices did not always show the exact onset of the dysrhythmia, so modern machines usually have a built in memory (60 seconds pre- and 60 seconds post-activation) which will hold the previously detected complexes. This increases the chances of picking up the start of the dysrhythmia, which is often very impor-tant for an accurate diagnosis.

2) Trans-telephonic recorders

These are small, hand-held solid-state recorders with electrodes affixed to the back. During an attack, the patient presses the unit firmly to the chest and a short rhythm sample is recorded (about 60 seconds). This may be transmitted as a modulated audio signal to a receiving station at the hospital (usually the coronary care unit) where the signal is decoded and printed out as a conventional ECG rhythm strip. The recorder can then be reset and used again. It is therefore very useful for infrequent, short-lived and recurrent symptoms.

3) Telemetric units

Telemetry is being used increasingly within hospitals for extended peri-infarction cardiac monitoring. The patient is fitted with standard chest electrodes attached to a small transmitter carried in a chest harness or pyjama pocket (see Figure 3.14). The cardiac rhythm is transmitted continuously to a receiver (normally situated on the cardiac care unit), where it is displayed, observed and analysed in the same way as the other patients on static monitors. The advantage of this system is that patients may be mobilised in the early period following myocardial infarction, whilst still having the benefits of dysrhythmia monitoring. The transmission range of these units is usually short, and thus relatively free from extrinsic radio interference. Longer range units have been developed for use by cardiac arrest teams within the hospital and by ambulance and paramedic teams outside the hospital. In both cases, the cardiac rhythm, and other parameters such as oxygen saturation may be monitored and transmitted back to the cardiac care unit so that advice on drug therapy can be given by more experienced physicians back at base.

Normal Variations seen on 24-hour Tapes

The heart rate varies throughout the day, being faster in the morning after waking, and then gradually slowing throughout the day to reach its slowest during sleep. Women have faster pulse rates than men by an average of about 5–10 beats per minute. As individuals grow older, the mean heart rate slows as does heart rate variability. Ectopic beats are very frequent, arising from both the atria and the ventricles, the latter being more common. Varying degrees of bradycardia and high atrio-ventricular block are often recorded in younger patients, particularly athletes; sinus pauses of 1.5 seconds are common, and pauses of up to 1.75 seconds are occasionally seen. Such findings are unlikely to be within normal limits in the elderly.

Recording Artifacts

Whichever recording system is used, artifactual interference is often encountered. Frequent causes include poor electrode contact, body movement and poor tape quality (due to tape stretch or inadequate tape erasure). Men with nylon shirts, or women with nylon underwear may also generate static electricity which can distort recordings. Such underwear should not be worn during ambulatory recording. Recording artifacts may be obvious during rhythm analysis, although many complexes may closely resemble rhythm abnormalities; careful examination of related rhythm strips is often required to demonstrate that the recording is artifactual and thus prevent inappropriate intervention. The simultaneous recording of two ECG channels is extremely helpful in this respect.

Common types of artifact include:

* Interference (movement, static) simulating ventricular tachycardia
* Disconnected or loose leads simulating asystole or pauses
* Variations in tape speed due to low batteries or stretched tape simulating bradycardias or tachycardias.

The Value of Ambulatory Monitoring

There are several major uses of ambulatory monitoring techniques:

1) Diagnosing the aetiology of symptoms

Confirmation of a rhythm induced diagnosis requires the concurrence of symptoms and a dysrhythmia. Asymptomatic recordings do not usually help, although evidence of asymptomatic abnormalities such as short runs of ventricular tachycardia or ischaemic *ST* segment abnormalities may help further management.

Approximately 60% of Holter recordings will show no abnormality, and a further 30% will be normal despite symptoms being documented during the recording period. A positive diagnosis is only made in 10% of cases where symptoms coincide with a dysrhythmia.

2) Assessment of the incidence and frequency of previously identified ischaemia or dysrhythmias

Rate dependent conduction disturbances or dysrhythmias caused by metabolic or ischaemic changes are often demonstrated this way. An increasing use is detection of silent myocardial ischaemia, since *ST* segment analysis is now considered to be more valid. A two-channel recorder is needed to record leads MCL-2 and MCL-5 simultaneously.

3) Immediate analysis of a dysrhythmia

By use of trans-telephonic or telemetric units, immediate rhythm analysis is available. This mode of monitoring is widely used for pacemaker function reports. In-patient telemetry also allows extended ambulatory monitoring of patients with recent myocardial infarction.

4) Assessment of anti-dysrhythmic therapy

Comparison of tapes before and after drug administration can help assess the efficacy of any chosen drug and give warning of pro-arrhythmia.

5) Assessment of patients following myocardial infarction and cardiac arrest

Continued myocardial irritability strongly associates with sudden cardiovascular death within the first year following acute myocardial infarction. Ventricular irritability can be determined by pre-discharge Holter monitoring, when the finding of complex ventricular dysrhythmias (ventricular tachycardia, multi-focal ectopics, etc.) may be an indication for early angiography. A full 24 hour recording is not normally required, and a 6 hour tape is usually adequate.

Continuous monitoring following cardiac arrest may demonstrate frequent ventricular extra-systoles, or short runs of ventricular tachycardia which may provide a guide for long-term prognosis and therapy. Advanced degrees of sino-atrial or atrio-ventricular block may also be documented during activity which may have been the underlying cause of the cardiac arrest.

6) More recent applications

With the technological advances over the last decade, powerful personal computers have expanded the traditional role of the Holter monitor. Such variables as ST segment monitoring, heart rate variability, QT interval measurement and signal averaged exercise electrocardiography can now be performed.

Chapter 7
An Introduction to Haemodynamic Monitoring

The term haemodynamic monitoring describes the monitoring of intra-vascular pressures, the blood volume and the blood circulation. This may be required to establish a precise diagnosis, or to determine the appropriate therapy for the condition or to monitor the effect of the chosen therapy. Most haemodynamic monitoring is achieved by the insertion of catheters into the heart or major blood vessels. The catheters are usually connected by fluid filled tubing to pressure transducers and recording systems, although miniature recorders can now be inserted directly into the circulation. The precise methods of obtaining and recording the haemodynamic status of the patient varies from hospital to hospital, and is usually dependent upon the expertise of the staff and available equipment. The extent of monitoring depends upon how much data is required to optimise the condition of the patient, and may be classified as:

a) *Non-invasive monitoring* – when there is no breech of the patient's skin

b) *Invasive monitoring* – when catheters and probes are introduced into the body

c) *Diagnostic monitoring* – monitoring required to make a diagnosis, for example, prior to cardiac surgery

d) *Derived monitoring* – when the variously recorded data are used to calculate other parameters derived from primary measurements, for example, measurement of peripheral resistance.

The most frequently measured haemodynamic parameters are the pulse rate, the arterial blood pressure, the central venous pressure (CVP), intra-cardiac pressures and the cardiac output. The most frequent derived parameters are the systemic and pulmonary vascular resistance.

Indications for Haemodynamic Monitoring

Patients who require haemodynamic monitoring usually have either problems with the heart or problems with the circulatory system, or both.

a) Problems with the heart

Essentially, the heart is little more than a mechanical pump. Conditions associated with 'pump failure' include acute myocardial infarction, ischaemic heart disease and cardiomyopathy. If the pump fails, there is a fall in cardiac output with decreased peripheral perfusion. Metabolic disorders (eg. acidaemia), and certain drugs may also be associated with cardio-depression, which will impair pump function.

b) Problems with the circulatory system

A fall in the circulatory volume will lead to circulatory failure. Such conditions include haemorrhage, prolonged vomiting and diarrhoea and diabetic keto-acidosis. Trauma, including surgery, may also produce profound fluid shifts within the body fluid compartments (eg. oedema) producing a fall in circulating volume.

Once a catheter has been inserted, patient comfort and safety, maintenance of the system and obtaining and recording data is usually a nursing responsibility. Since treatment will often rely heavily on the results of monitoring, it is essential that such data is accurate. This requires an awareness of the inherent problems in data acquisition, including common technical and physiological variables which may affect the readings. In addition, the effect in which specific nursing interventions (eg. feeding, bathing, positioning) may have on haemodynamic measurements and results will need consideration.

Pressure-Transducer Monitoring Systems

The measurement of intra-vascular and intra-cardiac pressures requires arterial or venous catheterisation. The catheter is either connected to fluid filled tubing and an external pressure transducer which connects electrically to the bedside monitor, or is an electronic catheter which has a micro-manometer at its tip and relays electrical signals externally.

The pressure monitor system therefore has three essential components: a transducer, an amplifier and a recorder.

a) The Transducer

Pressure transducers are electro-mechanical devices which detect energy changes, for example changes in pressure or changes in temperature, and converts them to electrical signals. In most forms of haemodynamic monitoring, they detect intra-vascular pressure changes and convert them into electrical charges which are subsequently amplified and recorded.

Pressure transducers are usually mounted externally. A wide variety of types are available, ranging from small units that attach to the arm, to bulky units which are kept beside the bed. Transducer holders enable the height at which the transducer lies to be varied, according to the zero reference point on the patient. Intra-vascular pressure changes are transmitted via fluid filled tubing to a supple diaphragm located in a fluid filled transducer dome (Figure 7.1). The changing pressure waves are directly transmitted to the diaphragm within the dome which is connected to a strain gauge. The more the diaphragm is moved by the pressure waves, the greater the electrical charge generated, and the higher the pressure reading on the monitor.

Disposable domes are more commonly in use now, and these preclude inaccuracy due to damage as well as the need for re-sterilisation.

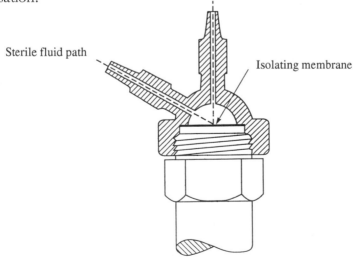

Sterile fluid path

Isolating membrane

Figure 7.1 The disposable fluid filled transducer dome. Sterile fluid from the pressure line passes over the isolating membrane which makes direct contact with the strain gauge and transducer

More recently, with miniaturisation, transducers which can fit into the proximal end of catheters have been designed. This precludes the need for fluid filled pressure tubing and increases the fidelity of the pressure recording. These special catheters may be advanced directly into the vessel concerned to measure not only pressure changes, but variations in acid–base balance or arterial blood gases.

b) The Amplifier

The signal amplifier is contained in the main monitor, and allows the electrical signal detected from the diaphragm to be amplified so that it may be displayed on the monitor screen. The amount of amplification required depends upon the pressure waves encountered. The system will therefore require calibration before use.

c) The Recorder

The amplified signal may be displayed either digitally as an analogue read-out, or graphically as a continuous waveform. The information may be utilised to derive haemodynamic parameters such as cardiac output, cardiac index, mean peripheral and pulmonary vascular resistance. With technical advances, internal computers may do this automatically from the accumulated data.

The Flushing System

A continuous flushing system is required to prevent clotting in the system, and normally employs a heparin/saline mixture infused at high pressure. A pressure infusion cuff compresses a bag containing the flushing solution to a pressure of about 300 mmHg. The normal flushing solution comprises 500 ml 0.9% saline with 500–1500 units of sodium heparin added. It should be set to run at 1–3 ml/hour.

Specialised connecting tubing is required to minimise distortion of the pressure wave signal. This connecting tubing is stiffened, high pressure tubing which prevents the pressure waves received from the in-dwelling catheter from being 'damped' (ie. smoothed). For the same reason, the length of tubing between the patient and the transducer should be as short as possible, and certainly less than four feet (120 cm).

Three-way taps may be incorporated into the infusion line to enable fluids to be withdrawn, diverted or aspirated as required. All ports not in use should be closed off with a suitable bung to preserve sterility and prevent the entry of air. To minimise the risk of infection, the flushing system and tubing should be replaced every 48–72 hours.

Preparation of the Transducer System

The following stages are required to prepare the transducer system:

a)   Heparin should be added to the infusion solution at a concentration of 1–3 units of heparin per millilitre of saline.

b)   The heparin solution is connected to a standard giving set, and the infusion bag is placed inside a pressure cuff. This cuff will be later inflated to 300 mmHg to maintain patency of the infusion line.

c)   The giving set is connected to the inflow port of the pressure valve which fits directly onto the pressure transducer and pressure dome.

d)   The transducer dome should be completely filled with fluid. No air bubbles must remain.

e)   A three-way tap is attached to the distal port of the pressure dome.

f)   An intra-venous extension plus a further three-way tap connects to the intra-vascular catheter after thorough flushing to remove all air from the system.

The assembled apparatus is shown in Figure 7.2.

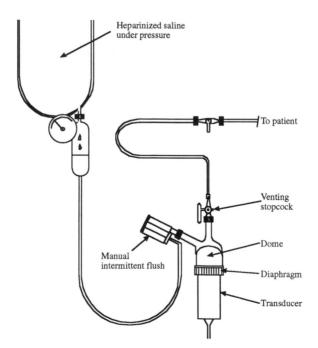

Heparinized saline
under pressure

To patient

Venting
stopcock

Manual
intermittent flush

Dome

Diaphragm

Transducer

Figure 7.2 The pressure-transducer system

Calibration

The pressure recording may be altered by the position of the patient or a changing atmospheric pressure. Baseline calibration and a constant reference point are required before monitoring can take place. It is advisable to delay zeroing of the system until last, so that the equipment has time to warm up and the temperature in the transducer has stabilised.

The first step is to ensure that all air bubbles throughout the system have been eliminated, and especially those within the transducer dome. The transducer is then placed at the proposed zero height and is then zeroed by opening it to air (ie. atmospheric pressure). This is assigned the zero reference point. It is essential that atmospheric pressure provides the baseline, and that subsequent pressure measurements are related to a constant reference point. The usual reference point on the patient is that which approximates to the position of the left atrium, a site known as the *phlebostatic axis*. This is located at the intersection of an imaginary plane passing longitudinally through the body in the mid-axillary line and a secondary transverse plane at the level of the 4th rib with the sternum (Figure 7.3). The phlebostatic axis should be marked on the patients chest to ensure pressure readings are taken with reference to the same zero point. The transducer is then located on the same level (the phlebostatic level), so that it remains in line with the height of the left atrium during pressure measurements.

Calibration is then required by giving the height of the recorded waveform a reference value. This is normally done by generating a pulse wave of known height, and setting the machine at a given value. For example, a 1 cm standard wave could be made to equate to 20 mmHg pressure recording. Calibration will depend upon which parameter is being measured. For example, venous lines may need to have a range of −20 to +50 mmHg. Arterial lines may need calibration up to 300 mmHg.

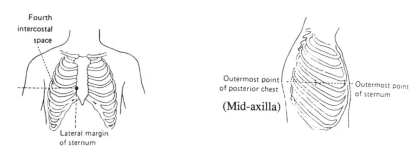

Figure 7.3 Landmarks of the phlebostatic axis

If the patient or the equipment is moved, the system should be re-calibrated, and this should be done anyway at least every eight hours.

Variation of Pressure Readings with Respiration and Body Position

The pressures in the heart and pulmonary circulation vary during the normal respiratory cycle, being lower on inspiration than on expiration. These changes predominantly affect the right side of the heart (being thin walled), and are also present during artificial ventilation, particularly with positive end-expiratory pressure (PEEP) and inspiratory mandatory ventilation (IMV).

Measuring haemodynamic pressures at end-expiration is considered to be the most valid, because the intra-thoracic pressure is closest to zero at this point. However, other methods of allowing for pressure variations through the respiratory cycle may include pressure averaging or simply reading the calculated mean pressure given on digital displays.

Reliable haemodynamic measurements may be obtained with the patient in a variety of different positions, provided a consistent technique is employed for each individual patient. The transducer should be at the phlebostatic level, regardless of the patient's position. If the transducer remains aligned with the phlebostatic level, measurement of pressures may take place with the head of the bed up to 45 degrees, which eliminates the need to lower the head of the bed each time a measurement is recorded. Transducers which are placed too high or too low record readings which are too low or too high respectively.

Use of Haemodynamic Monitoring Systems

Pressure-transducer monitoring systems are commonly used for:

a)   Central venous pressure monitoring
b)   Systemic arterial blood pressure monitoring
c)   Pulmonary artery blood pressure monitoring
d)   Mixed venous oxygen saturation monitoring.

Central venous pressure monitoring is very common in hospital practice. Whilst simple manometry, using a column of fluid, is the simple method of measuring the central venous pressure, it is preferable to utilise a pressure transducer system for greater accuracy. This is the preferred method in most high dependency units.

In seriously ill patients, indirect estimation is not only very difficult, but often very inaccurate. Direct determination of intra-arterial
pressure is usually needed to measure the systolic and diastolic blood
pressures reliably, and to calculate the mean arterial blood pressure
to ensure an adequate tissue perfusion pressure.

Right heart catheterisation with a four-channel pulmonary artery
catheter can be carried out at the bedside to determine intra-cardiac
pressures, including the central venous pressure, pulmonary arterial
pressures, wedge pressures and the cardiac output. Derived parameters include the stroke volume, the cardiac index and the systemic
and pulmonary vascular resistance.

Assessment of tissue metabolism, which is determined by the mixed-
venous oxygen saturation may be carried out intermittently via samples
taken through a pulmonary artery catheter, or continuously using a
pulmonary artery catheter fitted with a fibre-optic monitoring system.

Examples of Measured and Derived Haemodynamic Parameters

Clinical decisions about cardiac pre-load, afterload, contractility and
performance may be made from data obtained from monitoring
catheters, either from direct measurements, or from derived parameters derived from such data, as follows:

1) Central venous pressure = 2–6 mmHg

This is the filling pressure of the right ventricle (pre-load). It is measured
directly by a catheter in the superior vena cava or right atrium.

2) Pulmonary artery wedge pressure = 6–12 mmHg

This is an indirect measurement of the left atrial pressure, and
reflects the filling pressure of the left ventricle (left ventricular pre-
load). A catheter is sometimes inserted into the left atrium following
cardiac surgery to monitor this pressure, but more usually the left
atrial pressure is recorded indirectly by a pulmonary artery balloon
catheter (Swan-Ganz catheter) wedged in a pulmonary capillary.

3) Cardiac output = 4–6 litres/minute (at rest)

This is the volume of blood ejected by the left ventricle per minute. It
is measured by a thermodilution technique using a specific four-
channel pulmonary artery (Swan-Ganz) catheter.

4) Cardiac index = 2.2–4.0 litres/minute/m² (at rest)

This expresses the cardiac output relative to the size of the patient.

Many haemodynamic parameters are best expressed with regard to the patient's body surface area. The cardiac index is thus calculated by the cardiac output divided by the body surface area.

5) Stroke volume = 60–180 ml

The stroke volume is the amount of blood which the left ventricle ejects with each heart beat, and is an indication of left ventricular function. It is calculated by dividing the cardiac output (in ml) by the heart rate.

6) Systemic arterial blood pressures

Systolic = 100–140 mmHg
Diastolic = 70–90 mmHg
Mean = 70–115 mmHg

The systemic arterial blood pressure is most commonly measured indirectly using a mercury sphygmomanometer. Within hospital, an electronic (oscillometric) method is often utilised, whilst in high dependency areas, invasive monitoring via an indwelling arterial catheter is usual. Electronic methods will give the systolic, diastolic and mean arterial pressures as direct read-outs. Otherwise, the mean has to be calculated. The mean arterial blood pressure (MAP) is the average perfusion pressure created by the arterial blood pressure over one cardiac cycle. Since each cardiac cycle is roughly made up as one-third systolic timing and two-thirds diastolic timing, the calculation is:

$$\frac{(2 \text{ x diastolic blood pressure}) + \text{systolic blood pressure}}{3} \text{ mmHg}$$

7) Pulmonary arterial blood pressures

Systolic = 15–28 mmHg
Diastolic = 5–14 mmHg
Mean = 7–18 mmHg

These pressures are recorded by a pulmonary arterial catheter inserted directly into the pulmonary artery. Systolic and diastolic values are measured directly, and calculation of the mean pulmonary arterial pressure is automatic. Long-hand calculation is identical to that used for the mean systemic arterial blood pressure, ie.:

$$\frac{(2 \text{ x pulmonary diastolic pressure}) + \text{pulmonary systolic pressure}}{3}$$

8) Pulmonary vascular resistance (PVR) = 0.5–1.0 units or 40–80 dynes/second/cm⁵

This is the resistance against which the right ventricle must pump to eject blood. The resistance is caused by the pulmonary vasculature, although any resistance caused by the pulmonary valve must be taken into consideration. Normally, this is not significant, but may be in pulmonary stenosis. A raised PVR will reduce right-sided cardiac output and efficiency, whilst increasing right ventricular work and oxygen consumption.

The pulmonary vascular resistance is calculated by:

$$\frac{\text{Mean pulmonary arterial pressure} - \text{wedge pressure}}{\text{Cardiac output}} \text{ units}$$

Conversion to dynes/second/cm⁵ is made by multiplying units by 80.

9) Systemic vascular resistance (SVR) = 10–18 units or 800–1200 dynes/second/cm⁵

This is an index of the resistance against which the left ventricle must pump its volume. Resistance to left ventricular outflow is primarily due to arteriolar vasoconstriction. As for PVR, any degree of valvular obstruction (ie. aortic stenosis) must be taken into consideration.

Calculation of SVR is by:

$$\frac{\text{Mean arterial pressure} - \text{CVP}}{\text{Cardiac output}} \text{ units}$$

Conversion to dynes/second/cm⁵ is made by multiplying units by 80.

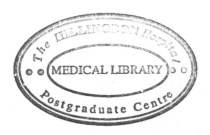

Chapter 8
Monitoring the Central Venous and Arterial Blood Pressure

Estimation of the central venous pressure (CVP) was one of the first techniques developed for haemodynamic monitoring, and measurement of the pressure of blood in the superior vena cava or right atrium is now commonly used in the assessment of cardiac function and intra-vascular volumes. Placement of CVP catheters is a frequent procedure on medical and surgical wards as well as intensive care areas. On the ward, measurement is usually intermittent via water manometers, whilst on critical care units, continuous monitoring using a pressure transducer with oscilloscopic display is more usual.

The Central Venous Pressure Wave

If a transducer and oscilloscope display are used, the venous waveform may be fully appreciated (Figure 8.1).

The *a* wave is produced by atrial contraction, and therefore follows the *P* wave on the ECG. If the atria do not contract, as in atrial fibrillation, no *a* wave is seen. Large *a* waves (cannon waves) may be seen if the right atrium contracts against a closed tricuspid valve. This may occur in tricuspid stenosis when the right atrial outlet is narrowed, or during complete heart block when contraction of the atria and ventricles are not synchronised.

The *a* wave is followed by the *x* descent which reflects the fall in pressure when the atria relax in diastole. It may merge with the *c* wave, which is caused by the tricuspid valve closing and then bulging back into the atrial cavity during ventricular contraction. It occurs after the *QRS* complex on the ECG.

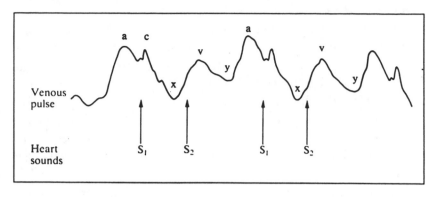

Figure 8.1 The venous pulse wave (From Jowett and Thompson: Comprehensive Coronary Care (2nd Ed) 1995. Reproduced by kind permission of Academic Press Ltd London)

The *v* wave records the pressure in the atrium during passive filling in diastole, which initially rises because the tricuspid valve is closed, and then falls when the valve opens. The *v* wave is followed by the *y* descent reflecting the fall in pressure as blood flows into the ventricles during ventricular diastole.

Indications for Monitoring the Central Venous Pressure

The major use of CVP measurement is for the assessment of the intra-vascular volume (Table 8.1). Assessing the CVP may additionally be utilised to give an indication of cardiac function, being an index of cardiac prc-load. The mean right atrial pressure (ie. CVP) correlates well with the right ventricular end-diastolic pressure, because when the tricuspid valve is open the right atrium and ventricle communicate and pressures equilibrate at the end of diastole. This then is an index of right ventricular pre-load.

Table 8.1: Some Indications for Inserting Central Venous Catheters

Following trauma or haemorrhage, when large volumes of intra-venous fluids are required

Post-operatively, particularly following major surgery

Patients requiring rehydration (eg. severe diarrhoea and vomiting, diabetic keto-acidosis)

Patients who are shocked

Patients with acute renal failure

For long-term intra-venous access (cytotoxic agents, antibiotic therapy, parenteral nutrition)

For calculation of the systemic vascular resistance* (SVR)

$$* \quad SVR = \frac{\text{Mean arterial pressure} - \text{CVP}}{\text{Cardiac output}}$$

Measuring the Central Venous Pressure

CVP catheters are inserted percutaneously, usually into the subclavian vein and advanced to lie in the superior vena cava or right
atrium. Other CVP cannula insertion sites include the median
basilic and the jugular veins. Although there are no valves between
the tricuspid valve and the vena cavae, the mean diastolic pressure is
a little higher in the vena cavae than in the right atrium (otherwise
blood would not flow). However for practical purposes, there is no
real difference in pressures recorded in either the superior vena cava
or the right atrium.

During central venous catheterisation, it is important that the
patient is placed in the Trendelenburg position (ie. head-down). This
distends the central veins, which not only reduces the risk of air-
embolism, but also makes cannulation easier. The right side of the
patient is chosen preferentially to prevent damage to the thoracic
duct. Placement is confirmed by chest X-ray, which will also exclude
the presence of an accidental pneumothorax. The line is normally
attached to a slow-running intravenous infusion and a manometer.

Positioning the patient is extremely important during measurement of the CVP. Ideally, the patient should be lying flat without a
pillow, but if the patient's condition does not permit this, they can be
positioned at 45 degrees or less, provided the zero point (normally
the phlebostatic axis) remains constant.

The pressure is normally measured using manometry, although
because of the sluggish response a pressure transducer system may
be preferred. This is particularly of value where continuous display
of the CVP is required. Although there is a little variation between
the systolic and diastolic right atrial pressures, the mean CVP is
usually recorded.

Manometry (Figure 8.2)

The manometer should be placed at the level of the right atrium (the
phlebostatic level). The baseline may be at zero on the scale, but it is
preferable to set it at a higher value (eg. 10 cm) so that negative pressures may be recorded. A spirit level should be used to ensure that
the zero reference point on both the patient and the manometer
coincide. The line should be flushed by opening up the intra-venous
fluid line. If this works smoothly, the CVP may then be measured.

The manometer column should be filled by turning the stopcock
from the normal position A to position B. The stopcock is then
turned to position C, and the fluid is then allowed to run down and
equilibrate through the CVP line. Normally the fluid falls freely,

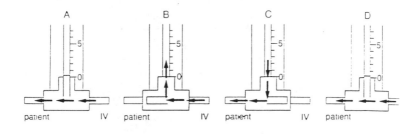

Figure 8.2 Monitoring central venous pressure. Proper stopcock positioning in a venous pressure manometer

although it fluctuates with venous pulsation and respiration. Once the column has settled, the CVP should be measured at the end of expiration, and expressed in cms H_2O (normal = 3–10 cms H_2O).

Following CVP measurement, the three-way tap should be returned to position A, and the infusion rate adjusted as required. It is important that the stopcock is adjusted to allow the infusion to continue, since the line may otherwise become occluded by clot. If intravenous fluids are being restricted, and the permitted intake is small, it is advisable to add a small amount of heparin to prevent clotting at slower infusion rates (0.5–1 unit heparin per millilitre of saline).

Pressure-transducer systems

This is most frequently utilised when measurements are made via the right atrial port of a four-channel pulmonary artery (Swan-Ganz) catheter, although dedicated lines may be connected directly to a pressure transducer. The pressure waveform is shown by continuous display and the reading recorded by the transducer is displayed in mmHg (normal = 2–6 mmHg).

Correlation of CVP in mmHg and cms H_2O is shown in Table 8.2.

If the patient is being ventilated (especially with positive end-expiratory pressure), a falsely high reading may be obtained. The most stable point of the respiratory cycle is end-expiration and readings taken at this point should be most reliable.

Problems with CVP Measurement

The CVP reading may be erroneous under the following circumstances:

1) Blocked cannula

The CVP will over-read. Free passage of fluid through the system should occur when the infusion rate is turned up and blood should

Table 8.2: Conversion of mmHg to cmsH₂O (approximate).

(mmHg x 0.36 = cms H₂O)	
1 = 1	11 = 15
2 = 3	12 = 16
3 = 4	13 = 18
4 = 5	14 = 19
5 = 7	15 = 20
6 = 8	16 = 22
7 = 10	17 = 23
8 = 11	18 = 24
9 = 12	19 = 26
10 = 14	20 = 27

Conversion of cms H_2O to mmHg = cms H_2O / 1.36

be freely aspirated if required. Respiratory oscillations should be visible during manometry.

2) Incorrect calibration

It is vitally important that pressure recordings are referrable to the level of the right atrium. Failure to adjust the position of the manometer after changing the patient's position is a common cause for incorrect CVP recordings.

If a transducer and oscilloscope are being used, they should be properly calibrated prior to use and frequently re-checked.

3) Catheter tip in wrong position

A check chest X-ray should always be taken to confirm the position of the catheter tip. It is not uncommon for over-long cannulae to enter the right ventricle, or for the catheter to migrate to this position with time.

4) Other infusions running through the CVP cannula

Other fluids are often infused through the same central line. Three-way taps or 'Y' connectors should not be in operation during CVP measurement. This is especially important when potent drugs such as dopamine are being infused. Flushing the CVP manometer may wash large quantities of the drug into the circulation, with possibly disastrous results.

Complications

The complications of CVP monitoring are similar to any situation where central venous catheterisation is employed (Table 8.3).

Table 8.3: Potential Complications of CVP Monitoring

---

a) During CVP insertion
       Pneumothorax
       Arterial puncture
       Malposition of catheter
       Air embolism
       Dysrhythmias
b) Early complications
       Extravasation of infusate
       Sepsis
       Delayed pneumothorax
       Subcutaneous emphysema
       Haemorrhage
c) Late complications
       Venus thrombosis
       Catheter related sepsis
       Air embolism

Infection at the catheter insertion site is common, especially from *Staphylococcus aureus, Staphylococcus epidermis* and the enterococci. This may occur at the time of insertion, or by subsequent colonisation by micro-organisms. The insertion site should be observed carefully for signs of inflammation. If infection occurs, the catheter must be removed, blood cultures taken through the line and the catheter tip sent for culture.

Malposition of the catheter is common, particularly following right subclavian vein puncture. The catheter commonly turns upwards into the neck veins and may cause the patient to feel pain in the side of the face. Alternatively the catheter may pass across into the left subclavian vein, or occasionally through the right ventricle and into the hepatic veins. Catheter position should always be checked with an X-ray.

Bleeding from the intravenous insertion site is uncommon, although there is an increased risk if the patient has a bleeding diathesis (ensure the platelet count is over $40,000 \times 10^9$ litre), has been taking anti-coagulants, or has just received coronary thrombolysis. If there has been difficulty in catheter placement, occult bleeding may occur and intra-thoracic bleeding may result in haemothorax or haemo-mediastinum.

Thromboembolic complications may occur if there has been stasis around the catheter tip; continual flushing of the system is desirable. Polyurethane catheters seem to be less irritant to the veins, and may be associated with a lower rate of thrombosis. Prophylactic heparin may minimise thrombotic complications.

Air embolism may occur if the line becomes disconnected; 100 ml of air can pass through a 14 gauge catheter every second, and as little as 10 ml or air may be fatal. A head-down (Trendelenberg) position should always be used during catheter insertion and removal, whilst dressings are being changed, or when tubing is being renewed.

If the catheter enters the right ventricle it usually gives rise to ventricular dysrhythmias due to irritation of the endocardium. Perforation of the right ventricle has been reported when inappropriately long catheters have been inserted.

Measuring the Blood Pressure

Blood pressure refers to the pressure within arteries as the heart pumps blood around the body, and is regulated by vasomotor tone in the arterial system, blood volume and cardiac output. The two pressures which are usually recorded are termed the systolic blood pressure and diastolic blood pressure. The systolic blood pressure (SBP) is the peak pressure recorded when the heart contracts and forces blood into the arterial system. The diastolic blood pressure (DBP) is that pressure recorded when the heart relaxes, and represents resting arterial tone. The arterial waveform may be seen during invasive monitoring techniques which demonstrate these systolic and diastolic components as a continuous waveform (Figure 8.3). The initial upstroke of the arterial pressure trace represents rapid ejection of blood into the major arteries following the opening of the aortic valve. This upstroke may be either exaggerated in patients with aortic incompetence and hyper-dynamic circulations (eg. pregnancy, thyrotoxicosis, fevers), or slowed in those with left ventricular failure or outflow obstruction (eg. aortic stenosis). As blood is distributed to the peripheries, the blood pressure falls until pressure in the left ventricle is less than that within the aortic root. The aortic valve then snaps shut, producing a characteristic 'dicrotic notch' in the descending waveform which marks the end of systole, and the beginning of diastole. As the blood flows to the peripheries, the pressure in the arterial system gradually falls until it reaches its lowest value – the diastolic pressure.

With invasive arterial monitoring, the configuration of the arterial waveform will vary, depending upon how close to the heart the pressure is measured. For example, the systolic pressures are higher and the waveform narrower if the catheter is in a peripheral artery. In addition, the dicrotic notch is less well seen. The actual systolic and diastolic blood pressures will also vary, although the mean arterial pressure will remain the same.

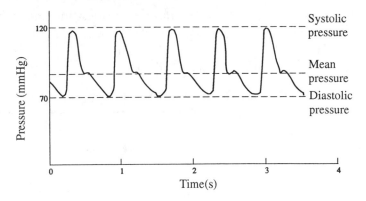

Figure 8.3 Arterial pulse wave

The pulmonary arterial pressure waveform is similar to the aortic arterial waveform, although the systolic peak in the pulmonary artery is only one-fifth of that in the aorta.

Mean Arterial Pressure (MAP)

The mean arterial pressure is not the sum of the systolic blood pressure plus the diastolic blood pressure divided by two. It is a measurement which gives the average perfusion pressure generated by the arterial blood pressure over the complete cardiac cycle (Figure 8.4). Since the cardiac cycle is approximately one-third systole, and two-thirds diastole, the mean arterial pressure is calculated by adding these three components:

$$MAP = 1/3\ SBP + 2/3\ DBP$$

or

$$MAP = \frac{SBP + (2 \times DBP)}{3}$$

This calculation is usually done automatically on modern electronic machines.

In patients with a low cardiac output, maintaining the mean arterial blood pressure above 50 mmHg will usually ensure adequate perfusion of the brain, kidneys and coronary arteries.

Units of Blood Pressure Measurement

The original units introduced by Poiseuille for the mercury manometer still persist, so that blood pressure continues to be measured in millimetres of mercury (mmHg). However, the International System of Units, adopted by many countries (including the UK) should have lead to replacement of mmHg by kilopascals (kPa), where 1 mmHg = 0.13 kPa, or 1 kPa = 7.52 mmHg.

A guide to conversion is shown in Table 8.4.

Table 8.4: Conversion Calculation for mmHg to kPa and Vice Versa

Converting mmHg to kPa	Converting kPa to mmHg
Double the pressure	Multiply the pressure by 10
Double it again	Divide by 2
Divide by 3	Divide by 2
Divide by 10	Multiply by 3

Hence, a blood pressure of 120/80 mmHg is roughly equivalent to 16/11 kPa.

As yet, the use of the kilopascals has not really caught on for routine blood pressure measurement, although it has done so for blood gas analysis in some hospitals.

Historical Methods of Measuring Blood Pressure

The first recorded measurement of blood pressure was in 1730, by the Reverend Stephen Hales who measured the height to which a column of blood reached when he inserted a glass tube into the neck veins of a horse. The tube had to be more than 8 feet long (240 cm)! Fortunately, Scipione Riva-Rocci devised the sphygmomanometer in 1896, which greatly cleaned up and simplified blood pressure estimation. Blood pressure is still most commonly measured indirectly with an aneroid or mercury sphygmomanometer, although precise measurement of arterial blood pressure requires a return to 'old-fashioned' intra-vascular monitoring.

The Riva-Rocci (auscultatory) method of blood pressure estimation employs a sphygmomanometer to occlude the brachial artery and a stethoscope to detect sounds of turbulent blood flow within the artery following the release of arterial compression. These sounds are known as the *Korotkoff sounds*, named after Nicholi Korotkoff, a Russian army surgeon who described them in 1905. Mercury sphygmomanometers are widely available in hospital practice and are more useful than the aneroid type which require frequent re-calibration. This auscultatory method of determining blood pressure has now been superseded in some modern machines by an oscillometric technique which employs a sensing pressure transducer to detect minute oscillations of the blood and vessel wall which start as the systolic pressure is reached, and continue until there is no arterial constriction.

Measuring Blood Pressure with a Mercury Sphygmomanometer

There are numerous factors which may lead to inaccurate assessment of the arterial blood pressure with the sphygmomanometer. It is surprising how many common errors are made by those who measure blood pressures every day. Some of these are made because the measurement is rushed and some because the proper technique has never been learned. The importance of accuracy is sometimes under-estimated as well; the person measuring the blood pressure may not be the one making decisions based on its measurement.

There are several steps which must be taken to minimise errors.

a) Preliminary

It is important that the equipment is checked thoroughly and regularly before being used for blood pressure measurement. Many pieces of equipment in daily use are in an unfit condition for the job. The mercury column must be at zero with the column vertical. The valve must move freely and not leak, and the cuff must be in good condition and of the correct size.

During blood pressure measurement, the sphygmomanometer mercury column must be vertical, and no more than three feet (90 cm) away from the observer so that it may be easily seen. The vertical scale must be able to be viewed straight on, with the eye at the level of the top of the mercury column. Resting the machine on the edge of the bed does not usually allow these factors, and it is surprising how often wall mounted equipment is in positions or heights which do not allow proper visibility.

Any clothing which prevents proper cuff application should be removed from the patient's upper arm, particularly if the sleeves are tight. If a pyjama jacket of shirt cannot be removed, it is better to place the cuff over the sleeve rather than causing a tight band by rolling the sleeve up.

b) Cuff and bladder size

The appropriate selection and application of the blood pressure cuff is very important, especially in children and obese patients. The cuff is the inelastic sleeve which encloses the bladder which will actually compress the arm. 'Cuff size' actually refers to the size of the bladder. The choice of cuff should be based upon the measurement of arm circumference, and clear marking of cuff bladder size by the manufacturers would be useful in this context. It is easy to be misled by terms such as 'paediatric cuffs'; the correct size is solely dependent upon arm circumference so that a big enough bladder is used.

A bladder which completely encircles the arm will give the most accurate results; if the bladder is too short, the blood pressure will be over-estimated. The bladder length should always be able to cover more than two-thirds of the circumference of the arm. Bladder lengths vary from around 22–36 cm.

The width of the cuff (and hence bladder) is also important. The recommended width is 20% greater than the diameter of the limb. This is equivalent to 40–50% of the mid-arm circumference (and certainly not less than 40%). A simple guide can be employed to show the best available cuff width based upon arm size (Figure 8.4). Cuffs which are too narrow will over-estimate the blood pressure.

Hence, the typical 'normal adult' bladder size should be about 13 × 35 cm. Once the correct cuff size is selected, it should be recorded, and the same size should always be used for serial measurements in the same patient.

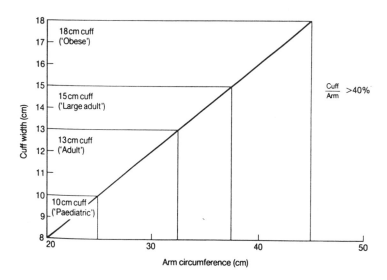

Figure 8.4 Blood pressure cuff sizes graph. This shows the correct blood pressure cuff (bladder) width based on the circumference of the patient's arm. The bladder sizes within each of the three commonly available cuff are shown (adult, large adult, obese adult). Note that the WIDTH of the bladder should be at least 40% of the arm circumference and the LENGTH of the bladder should encircle at least two-thirds of the arm.

c) Positioning the patient

The patient should be comfortable with the forearm supported, slightly extended and externally rotated. If the bladder does not completely encircle the arm, it must go more than two-thirds around with the centre of the bladder overlying the brachial artery. Most cuffs are usually marked to indicate the centre of the bladder which should be applied firmly and smoothly 2–3 cm above the ante-cubital fossa. In many patients, and especially if the arm is small, it may be easier to put the cuff on upside down so that the tubing points towards the patient's shoulder. This leaves the antecubital fossa well exposed for positioning of the stethoscope over the brachial artery.

The position of the patient is usually not important. Normally the diastolic blood pressure rises a little on standing, with a slight fall in the systolic blood pressure. There is little difference between sitting and lying blood pressure. However, in patients with auto-nomic failure, taking vasodilator medication or in shock, this fall may be very marked (postural or orthostatic hypotension). Record-ing supine and erect blood pressures is then of importance, and gives an indication of the integrity of the baro-receptor reflex. The position of the patient during blood pressure recording should always be recorded.

Whilst the position of the patient does not usually influence the blood pressure, the correct positioning of the arm is very important for accurate blood pressure assessment. There is a progressive increase in the systolic blood pressure of about 5 mmHg as the arm is moved down from the horizontal to the vertical when the patient is standing. The arm should always be positioned at the level of the heart. Additionally, if the arm is unsupported, isometric muscle contraction needed to hold the arm up against gravity can raise the diastolic blood pressure by up to 10%. This seems to be more marked in hypertensive patients, particular those taking beta-blockers. Hence, the arm should be supported horizontal with the nipples, either by resting on the desk if the patient is sitting, or by the observer physically supporting the arm if the patient is standing.

d) Cuff inflation

The cuff should firstly be inflated whilst feeling the brachial pulse until it can no longer be felt. This will give an approximation of the systolic pressure, and prevent under-estimation because of the auscultatory gap (see below). The cuff should then be fully deflated to allow the veins to empty, and then re-inflated to approximately 30 mmHg above the previously determined systolic blood pressure. The mercury column should be observed at eye-level and allowed to fall at 2–3 mm/second by careful control of the valve. Faster or slower rates of deflation may lead to inaccurate readings.

Venous congestion must be avoided, so the cuff should be inflated as quickly as possible and deflated completely between successive readings. Prolonged inflation of the cuff is the most common cause of venous congestion which may raise the systolic blood pressure by 30 mmHg above or 15 mmHg below the actual systolic pressure. There is a similar but smaller effect on the diastolic pressure. A suitable gap should take place between successive blood pressure readings to allow venous emptying.

e) Recording the blood pressure

The mercury column is allowed to fall slowly until a faint tapping sound is heard through the stethoscope which is applied firmly over the brachial artery. Whilst the bell of the stethoscope is better for detecting this sound, it is sometimes harder to maintain this in contact with the patient's arm with one hand and the diaphragm is more often employed. The first sounds heard equate to phase 1 of the Korotkoff sounds and is equivalent to the systolic blood pressure. It should be recorded to the nearest 2 mmHg. As the mercury column continues to fall, there is often a silent gap (phase 2) until the sounds are heard again (phase 3). The sounds then become faint (phase 4) until they disappear completely (phase 5). Both phase 4 and phase 5 have been used in the past as an indication of diastolic blood pressure. These days, phase 5 should be used universally (except in children), unless sounds are heard down to zero. In this instance, both the phase 4 and phase 5 blood pressure should be recorded (eg. 140/80/0 mmHg).

The arm used for recording should be noted, and initially the pressure in both arms should be recorded. There is usually a small difference in blood pressure between the arms, the right arm usually being higher by between 2–10 mmHg. Blood pressure should always be taken in the arm with the higher value if the difference is greater than 10 mmHg.

The full record should ideally include the systolic and diastolic blood pressures (with phase 4 or 5 recorded if appropriate), the arm used, the position of the patient, and the presence of any influencing factor (pain, stress, dysrhythmia). Attention to such details may make this routine procedure more valuable.

Systolic blood pressures recorded by palpation only should be marked with a 'P' (eg. 120/P), and via a Doppler probe with a 'D' (eg. 120/D).

Reasons for Error in Blood Pressure Estimation

1) Observer error and bias

Most observers record the blood pressure in values ending with a zero or five. This digital preference may lead to inaccuracies. It is recommended that blood pressure is recorded to the nearest 2 mmHg.

Behavioural influences also exert subtle but often important variance. Men have higher blood pressures when recorded by a woman. For women the reverse is true. Additionally, having your blood pressure taken by someone from a different racial background can falsely elevate the blood pressure.

There is a tendency for people to rush blood pressure estimation. If hurried, attention to detail is lost. The blood pressure cuff is often released too quickly, which leads to underestimation of the systolic blood pressure and overestimation of the diastolic blood pressure. If interrupted, exact figures may be forgotten and later estimated. It is important to write the figures down as soon as possible to avoid this. It is usual to record the blood pressure twice, using the second recording only to minimise observer error. A pause of two minutes should be left before the second estimation to allow the release of venous blood.

2) The auscultatory gap

In some patients there is a loss and reappearance of the Korotkoff sounds during cuff deflation in the latter part of phases 1 and 2, which may cover as much as 40 mmHg. It is particularly common in patients with high blood pressure and in patients with reduced arterial flow (low cardiac output or atherosclerotic vessels). If this is not recognised, spuriously high diastolic blood pressures will be recorded or the true systolic blood pressure will be missed. Inflating the cuff whilst palpating the artery in the first instance should eliminate this. Cardiac dysrhythmias, especially atrial fibrillation, may give variable beat to beat readings and provides a trap for the unwary. An average of several estimations is then required.

3) Technical error

Faulty and poorly maintained equipment may give rise to error. Common faults include leaking from the rubber tubing, air holes, faulty valves and leakage of mercury. The cuffs also become very worn, particularly those with Velcro fixing. With time, these tend to lose their grip, and the cuff will give way during inflation. Any cuff which does this should be discarded. Aneroid sphygmomanometers have been shown to be particularly temperamental and need frequent re-calibration. They are best avoided.

There are certain occasions when blood pressure estimation is difficult. This is particularly so in severe hypotension, when indirect readings with the mercury sphygmomanometer are inaccurate, and the Korotkoff sounds may not even be generated. Doppler detection or invasive monitoring techniques are then required (see below).

Doppler Determination of Blood Pressure

Christian Doppler, an Austrian physicist, first described the phenomenon which may be observed by listening to the high pitched sound as a train approaches, which then changes to a low pitched sound as it travels away (the Doppler phase shift). The Doppler principle is widely used in vascular studies by directing ultrasonic sound waves at moving red cells, and recording the reflected sound. High frequency Doppler probes (6–10 MHz) will detect these returning sound waves in vessels close to the skin to produce an audible signal which represents blood flow through the vessel. Doppler probes may be used to replace the stethoscope for measuring systolic blood pressure more accurately in hypotensive patients and where there is a high systemic vascular resistance. The probe (with conducting gel) is placed over the brachial or radial artery and used to detect arterial flow as the sphygmomanometer cuff is deflated.

Electronic blood pressure machines using the Doppler technique have a probe placed under the sphygmomanometer cuff. The systolic blood pressure is picked up as soon as red cell flow is detected, and the diastolic blood pressure is recorded at the point when it starts to diminish.

Automatic and Semi-automatic Blood Pressure Recorders

Over the last few years, many automated blood pressure measuring devices have appeared. Some employ a microphone which is positioned over the brachial artery to detect the Korotkoff sounds, whilst others work by oscillometry or Doppler ultrasound. Oscillometric systems have shown themselves to be particularly useful and can efficiently measure systolic, diastolic and mean blood pressures (eg. Dinamap, Critikon Ltd, Berkshire – Figure 8.5). Such machines are now widely utilised in high dependency areas. Arterial pulsations are transmitted via the whole cuff, not a microphone, and hence precise

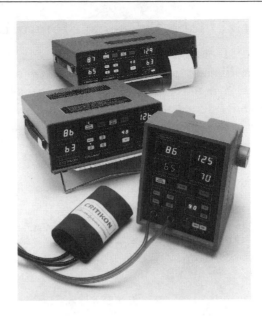

Figure 8.5 Dinamap Oscillometric blood pressure recorders (Reproduced by kind permission of Critikon Ltd, Berkshire)

location of the cuff over the artery is not required. It can even measure blood pressure through shirt sleeves! The oscillations start at the systolic pressure and continue below the diastolic pressure with the point of maximum oscillation corresponding to the mean intra-arterial pressure. Because these end points are not accurate, special electronic circuitry allows indirect calculation with improved accuracy. The machine has a motion-artifact rejection system, such that only when two identical pulses are found will the cuff deflate further. If there has been any external movement or vibration artifact, this will be eliminated. Typically, readings take less than half a minute, and an automatic cycle mode allows repeated measurements to be made at intervals of between 1 and 90 minutes. The machine will display pulse rate, systolic, diastolic and mean arterial blood pressure.

Miniature portable recorders using a oscillometric finger cuff are available, but not very accurate.

With oscillometric devices, it is important that a correct cuff size is employed and that it fits snugly around the arm. In obese patients, where the upper arm may be cone shaped, the forearm or ankle may be a better choice. The machines need regular calibration, and adherence to the service contract schedule is desirable.

In very hypotensive or unstable patients, the recordings may be inaccurate and invasive blood pressure monitoring is then recommended.

Intra-arterial Blood Pressure Monitoring

In the unstable patient, indirect measurement of the blood pressure is not only very difficult but may be very inaccurate, particularly if there is marked hypotension. In shock, readings taken in this way may differ from the actual arterial blood pressure by over 30 mmHg. The insertion of an arterial pressure line is useful for directly and continuously measuring systolic, diastolic and mean arterial blood pressures, as well as for giving easy access for repeated arterial blood sampling. Some indications for arterial pressure monitoring are shown in Table 8.5.

Table 8.5: Some Indications for Invasive Blood Pressure Monitoring

Intensive care patients
Major cardio-thoracic and arterial surgery
Major neurosurgery
Operations where there may be sudden or profound blood loss
During induced hypotension

Sites commonly employed for cannula insertion are the radial, brachial and dorsalis pedis arteries. However, the closer the cannula is to the heart, the more accurate the waveform and the pressure reading. The most usual site therefore is the radial artery of the non-dominant hand as access and fixation are straightforward and collateral circulation is good since the ulnar artery is responsible for most of the hand's perfusion in the majority of people.

If cannulation of the radial artery is contemplated, then the integrity of the ulnar artery and collateral supply to the hand should be tested. This is done by the Allen test, although it must be noted that it is not infallible.

The Allen Test

The patient's hand is elevated to drain blood out which may be aided by the patient squeezing his hand. The radial and ulnar arteries are then compressed to shut off arterial blood supply to the hand. The hand is then relaxed and hung downwards. The ulnar artery is then released, whereupon the hand should recolour within 5–10 seconds. If this takes longer, the ulnar collateral circulation is inadequate and radial cannulation should not be attempted.

Cannulation

Cannulation is performed percutaneously under local anaesthesia, using a 20 gauge Teflon catheter (22 gauge for children). Larger catheters are more likely to cause thrombosis and occlusion. Parallel-sided cannulae should be chosen, since they allow blood flow to continue around the cannula once inserted. The catheter is secured with tape, a suture or both, and attached to a 'T' connector and pressurised saline/heparin flushing system. The 'T' connector allows arterial blood sampling, if required.

Localised thrombosis may affect up to a fifth of all cases although the majority re-cannalise when the cannula is removed. Thrombosis may be minimised if a saline/heparin flushing solution is allowed to run continuously at about 3–5 mls/hour. This will also reduce vasospasm and damage to the arterial intima. The system is maintained by a pressurised bag containing 1–4 units of heparin per millilitre of 5% dextrose. The pressure applied to the bag must of course be at a higher pressure than the systolic blood pressure to prevent reflux. A transducer is connected to the monitor which converts the recorded pressures into a continuous display of the arterial waveform with digital readout of the calculated systolic, diastolic and mean blood pressures.

The arterial waveform should show a sharp upstroke, then a gradual downstroke with a dicrotic notch when the aortic valve closes (see Figure 8.3). A damped waveform may indicate kinks or leaks in the system, partial occlusion by thrombus, air bubbles or occlusion of the catheter tip if, for example, the wrist is bent. If thrombus formation is suspected, it is good practice to gently aspirate 2–3 ml of arterial blood first to remove any fresh thrombus at the catheter tip, or embolisation may occur. To prevent damping from the effect of sludging of blood elements at the catheter tip, the line should have a rapid flush via a Sorenson Intraflow device which delivers a few millimetres of heparinised solution rapidly through the cannula every 1–2 hours. Another frequent cause of damping is air bubbles in the connecting system. These lodge in the pressure-transducer dome or the central hub of the three-way tap. They may also be removed by flushing or gentle tapping with the finger.

A damped arterial trace results in a recorded systolic pressure of less than it actually is. Indirect measurement with a traditional mercury sphygmomanometer from time to time is good practice to cross check the intra-arterial measurement system. Regular examination of the cannulated hand is required to ensure no ischaemic damage.

Other sources of error are shown in Table 8.6.

Table 8.6: Some Sources of Error and Artifact During Intra-arterial Blood Pressure Monitoring

---

1) Improper calibration
   Although modern pressure amplifiers incorporate an electrical calibration signal, its accuracy should always be checked against a mercury sphygmomanometer.

2) Equipment not zeroed
   Many types of monitor require frequent re-zeroing, particularly after the patient has moved, or sometimes following blood sampling.

3) Over or under-damping
   The introduction of small amounts of blood or air into the pressure tubing may have a major damping effect on the pressure tracing, particularly if blood samples are taken via the cannula.

4) Catheter tip occlusion
   Partial occlusion by thrombus will affect pressure readings.

Obtaining Arterial Blood samples from the Arterial Catheter

Arterial blood samples may be obtained via the 'T' connector. About 3–5 ml should firstly be drawn off and discarded since this will contain a mixture of blood and flush solution. The stopcock should be turned off to all ports before this syringe is removed. Another fresh heparinised syringe is then attached, and the stopcock turned to the arterial line for the sample to be taken. The stopcock is then turned again to exclude the sample port, and flushed rapidly for 2–3 seconds from the flush system. The sample port should also be flushed with a heparinised solution to prevent clots and infection resulting from blood retained in the hub. This may be done by holding gauze over the port and employing the flush system with the arterial port turned off.

Some machines require re-zeroing following blood sampling, and it is worth checking this before further arterial pressure measurements are recorded.

Complications

Complications of intra-arterial monitoring are not common, but include:

– occlusion (including spasm) leading to ischaemia
– haemorrhage
– air embolism
– bruising
– sepsis.

a) Obstruction

Local obstruction may cause distal ischaemia, which may be worsened if the patient is already peripherally hypo-perfused. The incidence of thrombosis is higher in patients who are critically ill, because of blood hyper-coagulability. Emboli may be seeded from primary thrombus at the catheter tip, or from dried blood in the stopcock and connecting tubing, if not cleared following arterial blood sampling.

The skin distal to the arterial puncture site requires regular inspection for signs of impaired perfusion. Medications should never be injected into the arterial line, or vasospasm may be precipitated resulting in distal gangrene.

b) Haemorrhage

If the pressure line becomes disconnected from the cannula, accidental blood loss of approximately 50 ml/minute may be anticipated. Hence, great care is required to ensure all connections are firmly in place. Many arterial pressure monitors have alarm systems which sound if a large or sudden pressure fall is recorded.

When the line is removed, pressure over the arterial puncture site should be maintained for at least 5 minutes, or longer if there are coagulation problems.

c) Sepsis

The dressing at the site of arterial puncture should be inspected and replaced daily. The tubing and flush solution should be renewed every 24 hours.

If there are signs of infection, the line should be removed immediately and the tip sent for culture. The site should also be swabbed and cultured.

d) Air embolism

The infusion and tubing must be kept free from bubbles. The drip chamber is a potential source of air embolism when the flush solution is allowed to pass through at high velocity.

Ambulatory Blood Pressure Measurement

Blood pressure is extremely variable, depending upon physical activity, emotional status, posture and other factors. The difference between the highest and lowest blood pressures recorded may be as much as 35 mmHg. The standard deviation of all readings is about plus or minus 10 mmHg. Nocturnal blood pressure readings are usually lower, probably relating to sleep rather than circadian variation. Blood pressure variability and daily profiles may be more important in defining the patient's cardiovascular risk, and those who do not drop their blood pressure during sleeping hours may accumulate more cardiovascular damage than those who do. Blood pressure readings in hospital or in the surgery may be higher than normal for that individual patient because of so-called 'white coat hypertension' (elevation of the blood pressure induced by medical consultation). Patient's home recordings are nearly always lower than those recorded in a medical environment. It may still be too early to know what relevance this has to our clinical practice, since it may be the hypertensive ('stress') peaks that relate more closely to cardiovascular risk.

Many portable devices are now available which can measure the blood pressure in ambulatory patients. Whilst it is possible to monitor the blood pressure continuously by the insertion of an arterial cannula attached to an ambulatory monitor, this is clearly not practical in studying the majority of patients.

Major advances in technology have resulted in a number of fully automatic, lightweight, non-invasive machines which take blood pressure utilising a normal blood pressure cuff which is inflated intermittently. These machines either employ a microphone which is positioned over the brachial artery to detect the Korotkoff sounds, or work by oscillometry. Devices using the oscillometric technique are simpler to use, and are more widely used in clinical practice. Machines which utilise detection of the Korotkoff sounds are more complex to implement. The microphone usually forms an integral part of the cuff which can cause problems if the cuff slips during exercise. Cleaning the microphone to ensure a good signal may also be a problem. Better reception is achieved if the microphone is separate and can be taped directly over the brachial artery. To improve accuracy, the machines can be co-wired with an ambulatory ECG signal from chest leads, thus ensuring that the microphone only picks up genuine arterial sounds.

The power pack contains batteries and a small computer so that the machine can be programmed to take serial blood pressure readings at pre-determined intervals. Usually 50–100 readings are taken per 24 hour sample period, the cuff being inflated automatically by a small pump or carbon-dioxide cylinder. The blood pressure readings are stored in the memory of the recorder, and can be down-loaded into a personal computer. It is usual to ask the patients to keep an activity diary through the day, since many variables such as eating, stress, exercise and posture may have marked effects on the recorded blood pressure.

The technique is subject to many errors, other than mechanical breakdown, and very few machines satisfy the validation criteria of the British Hypertension Society. Not many devices give good results during exercise, so a short buzzer can be made to sound before blood pressure measurement allowing the patient to straighten his arm at his side. This is particularly important during vigorous activity, or when in contact with vibrating apparatus. Variability in the position of the arm during recording may cause major discrepancies. In the day, the patient should be told to keep the arm parallel to the trunk, but night-time readings remain a problem if the patient lies on his or her side, when the recording arm will either be above the heart, or below the heart. This may vary the blood pressure by plus or minus 10 mmHg.

All non-invasive blood pressure machines estimate the systolic blood pressure with greater accuracy than the diastolic blood pressure. The results seem to produce lower figures than hospital recorded values, though not as low as self-measured home values. No currently available monitor works in all patients; the elderly and the obese seem to generate the most problems.

On the whole, ambulatory devices are reasonably accurate, and usually provide reproducible recordings. Machines which have not been validated by the British Hypertension Society or the American based Association for the Advancement of Medical Instrumentation should not be used.

Some Indications for Ambulatory Blood Pressure Monitoring

There are several circumstances where ambulatory blood pressure monitoring may be of value:

1) Evaluating the need for treatment in a newly diagnosed hypertensive patient without target organ damage
2) Evaluation of the efficacy of treatment of hypertension
3) In the investigation of labile hypertension
4) Where there is a great disparity between hospital, GP and home readings ('white coat hypertension')
5) In the assessment of orthostatic (postural) hypotension.

Analysing 24 hour Blood Pressure Recordings

The major current problem is evaluation of the recordings which is not straightforward. There are conflicting views on the place of ambulatory blood pressure monitoring in clinical practice. The best way to analyse the data from recordings is not known, and there is as yet no consensus on the normal ranges and thresholds for treatment based on ambulatory readings.

Several population studies of ambulatory blood pressure are now available which may allow us to define 'normality'. These studies suggest that daytime figures in excess of 155/95 mmHg are probably abnormal, and below 135/85 mmHg should be viewed as normal. The intermediate zone may be considered abnormal or normal, depending upon the patient's cardiovascular risk-factor profile.

For simple evaluation of the known hypertensive patient, the daytime recordings or 24 hour average recording is probably of most value. Those patients who are shown not to reduce blood pressures through the night may have secondary hypertension, and perhaps should be investigated more completely, although some patients with essential hypertension have this pattern.

Chapter 9
Haemodynamic Monitoring with Pulmonary Artery Catheters

Although monitoring heart rate, arterial blood pressure and central venous pressure provide a valuable guide to cardiovascular status, they often do not supply enough information for complete diagnosis, or for planning appropriate management. For example, the value of central venous pressure monitoring is limited because it only reflects the functional state of the right ventricle, which does not always parallel that of the left ventricle. Information about left ventricular performance is often essential for complete evaluation. This information may be acquired by the insertion of a pulmonary artery catheter, which will not only provide information about pulmonary vascular pressures, but can additionally provide information about left ventricular function by measurement of the pulmonary artery wedge pressure which is an index of left ventricular pre-load.

Many types of pulmonary artery catheters are available, the best known being the balloon tipped, flow directed Swan-Ganz catheter.

The Swan-Ganz Catheter

The Swan-Ganz catheter is named after Howard Swan and William Ganz who designed and reported its use in 1970. The catheter is about 80–110 cm in length, marked with black bands at 10 cm intervals, and is presented in three sizes: 5FG (for children), 6FG and 7FG (for adults). The basic model has two lumina. The larger lumen terminates at the tip of the catheter and is used for recording intra-cardiac pressures, infusion of fluids and sampling of mixed venous

145

blood. A smaller lumen provides a channel for inflation of the latex balloon at the tip of the catheter. When inflated it allows the catheter to float through the heart to measure pressures in the different chambers and to permit repeated, reversible pulmonary capillary occlusion for recording the pulmonary artery wedge pressure (PAWP). In more advanced designs, there is a third lumen terminating 30 cm proximal to the catheter tip, which enables simultaneous measurement of the right atrial pressure (ie.the CVP), and probably the most commonly utilised model is the four-channel Swan-Ganz catheter which has a thermistor located 4–6 cm proximal to the tip (Figure 9.1). This is utilised in the measurement of the cardiac output by a thermodilution technique.

Other models are available for pulmonary angiography and temporary endocardial pacing, and all may be floated into the correct location by observation of the intra-cardiac pressure waves as the catheter passes through the heart. Since fluoroscopy is not required, the Swan-Ganz catheter can be inserted at the bedside under local anaesthesia via central or peripheral veins, without needing to move the patient to a catheter laboratory or pacing room.

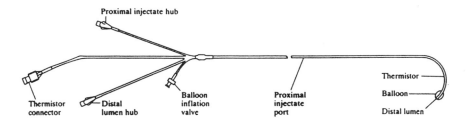

Figure 9.1 The Swan-Ganz catheter (From Stokes and Jowett, 1995. Reproduced by kind permission of Churchill Livingstone)

Pressure Recorded During Catheter Insertion

As the catheter is inserted, observation of the black surface markings enables the approximate position of the tip to be assessed. For example, the right ventricle lies approximately 20–25 cm from a right subclavian insertion site. Observation of the intra-cardiac pressure waves displayed on the bedside monitor enables more precise localisation of the catheter.

When inserted from the jugular or subclavian veins, the catheter enters the right atrium (RA) via the superior vena cava, and produces the waveform shown in Figure 9.2, with typical *a* and *v* waves of the venous pulse. Normal pressures in the RA vary between 2–6 mmHg, but should be measured as a 'mean' pressure which reflects the mean RA filling pressure (equivalent to the CVP). In the absence of significant tricuspid obstruction this is equivalent to the right ventricular end-diastolic pressure (RVEDP). A rise in the right atrial pressure may signal volume overload, right or left ventricular failure or pulmonary hypertension. High RA pressures are also found in patients with tricuspid valve disease or with cardiac tamponade.

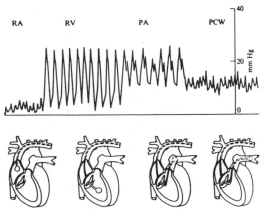

Figure 9.2 Pressure traces obtained during insertion of the Swanz-Ganz catheter (From Stokes and Jowett, 1995. Reproduced by kind permission of Churchill Livingstone)

Having recorded pressures in the right atrium, the latex balloon is inflated and the catheter is allowed to float through the tricuspid valve into the right ventricle. When this occurs, the pressure trace immediately changes as this high pressure area is encountered. Right ventricular systolic pressures vary from about 20–30 mmHg, with diastolic pressures similar to those in the right atrium (2–6 mmHg). The waveform appears as a large spike produced by iso-volumetric contraction of the right ventricle, which is followed by a fast downstroke as the pulmonary valve opens, the lowest point of the waveform representing the RVEDP (Figure 9.2). The pressure wave then climbs slowly upward as the right ventricle fills passively with blood from the right atrium. Right ventricular pressures are raised in the presence of increased pulmonary vascular resistance, or where there is increased pulmonary blood flow.

As the catheter passes through the pulmonary valve, there is little change in the systolic pressure, but the diastolic pressure rises, such that the amplitude of the waveform is reduced (Figure 9.2). The waveform shows a sharp upstroke with a gradual downstroke with a dicrotic notch caused by closure of the pulmonary valve. Systolic pressures here are normally between 20–30 mmHg with diastolic pressures lying between 10–12 mmHg. The diastolic pressure is approximately equal to the left atrial pressure unless the vascular resistance is elevated, and is equivalent to the left ventricular end-diastolic pressure (LVEDP). The mean PA pressure is automatically calculated by the monitor:

Mean PA pressure =   1/3 Pulmonary systolic pressure (PSBP) +
                                   2/3 Pulmonary diastolic pressure (PDBP)

                                             or

                                   PSBP + (2 x PDBP)
Mean PA pressure =   ─────────────────────────

                                             3

The mean pressure in the pulmonary artery reflects the combined effect of changes in the pulmonary vascular resistance (PVR) and pulmonary blood flow (right ventricular cardiac output). The relationship may be shown by:

$$\text{Pulmonary vascular resistance (PVR)} = \frac{\text{Mean PA pressure} - \text{PAWP}}{\text{Cardiac output}} \text{ units}$$

Conversion to dynes/second/cm^5 is made by multiplying units by 80. (Normal ranges = 0.5–1.0 units or 40–80 dynes/second/cm^5.)

Elevated PA pressures may be found when pulmonary blood flow is increased (eg. fluid overload, left ventricular failure, mitral stenosis) or when pulmonary vascular resistance is increased as in pulmonary hypertension, pulmonary embolism).

When the catheter tip reaches a pulmonary artery capillary smaller than the diameter of the balloon, it becomes wedged. In this position, the catheter will record pressure transmitted directly upon its tip – the pulmonary artery wedge pressure (PAWP). Since the pulmonary arteries are end-arteries (there are no pulmonary arterioles), and the pulmonary veins contain no valves, there is an unrestricted channel between the end of the catheter through to the left atrium, and thus the pressure here is recorded as the pressure wave travels through the continuous vascular channel to the catheter tip. It can be seen then, that the PAWP is actually an indirect recording of the left atrial pressure, and when the mitral valve opens, it can even be used to measure the left ventricular end-diastolic pressures (LVEDP). The PAWP ranges from 6–12 mmHg in the normal patient, which is nearly the same as the PA end-diastolic pressure in most cases (Figure 9.2). A gradient of more than 5 mmHg between the PAEDP and the wedge pressure is abnormal, and reflects increased pulmonary vascular resistance.

Provided the pulmonary vascular resistance is not too high (ie. PAEDP and PAWP differ by < 5 mmHg), the PAEDP may be utilised instead of the PAWP in many cases during treatment with drugs and fluids. Since the PAEDP is recorded continuously by the bedside monitor, using this value often precludes the need for multiple re-wedging of the catheter.

The PA pressure waveform should return promptly on deflation of the balloon, when elastic recoil returns the catheter tip into the main pulmonary artery. Occasionally, it is necessary to physically withdraw the catheter a little, to clear the narrow vessels. If the waveform is damped, it is due either to accumulation of small clots in the catheter, or alternatively because the tip may still not have been pulled far enough back into the pulmonary artery. In this case the catheter must be manually withdrawn a few more centimetres and the waveform inspected. If the waveform is still damped, the system should be 'fast flushed' to remove any debris away from the tip. On stopping the fast flush, the normal PA waveform should appear rapidly and completely.

Uses of the Swan-Ganz Catheter

The four-channel PA catheter is able to measure all the right heart pressures as shown in Table 9.1, plus the cardiac output.

Table 9.1: Normal Pressures in the Right Heart and Pulmonary Vessels

	Pressure (mmHg)
Right atrium	2 – 6
Right ventricle	
Systolic	15 – 28
Diastolic	1 – 6
Pulmonary artery	
Systolic	15 – 28
Diastolic	5 – 14
Mean	7 – 18
Pulmonary artery wedge	6 – 12

The Pulmonary Artery Wedge Pressure

The major value of the Swan-Ganz catheter is that by assessing the pulmonary artery wedge pressure it allows an indirect measurement of the left atrial pressure. In the normal heart, there is a predictable relationship between left atrial and right atrial pressures. However, in critically ill patients this is not always the case, and knowledge of the left atrial pressure is often of great importance. Obtaining a left atrial pressure directly would either involve cardiac puncture, or retrograde passage of an aortic catheter, but fortunately the pressure recorded by the Swan-Ganz catheter wedged in a pulmonary capillary is equivalent to that in the left atrium. Knowledge of the left atrial pressure is of value in deciding whether pulmonary oedema has a cardiac or non-cardiac aetiology.

As the left atrial pressure (LAP) rises it causes exudation of fluid out of the pulmonary vasculature and into the interstitial and intra-alveolar spaces to produce pulmonary oedema. Typically, an LAP of 20 mmHg marks the onset of pulmonary congestion and above 25 mmHg there is obvious pulmonary oedema. Pulmonary oedema in the presence of a low wedge pressure is a feature of the adult respiratory distress syndrome (ARDS).

The adult respiratory distress syndrome describes respiratory failure which usually arises from a non-respiratory pathology which does not directly affect the lung, such as sepsis, major trauma, haemorrhage or burns. It commonly associates with failure of the other vital organs, either singly or as part of the multiple organ failure syndrome. The criteria for the diagnosis of ARDS are shown in Table 9.2.

Table 9.2: Criteria for the Diagnosis of the ARDS

- Refractory hypoxaemia (arterial oxygen tension < 8 kPa) despite 40% oxygen and positive end-expiratory pressure > 5 cm H_2O)
- Bilateral pulmonary infiltrates seen on the chest X-ray, suggestive of pulmonary oedema
- Normal or low PA wedge pressure
- 'Stiff lungs'

Monitoring Patients with the Respiratory Distress Syndrome

ARDS is associated with increased peripheral oxygen consumption, a low mixed venous oxygen saturation (SVO_2), and variable left atrial pressures. The condition therefore requires insertion of a four-channel PA catheter to allow measurement of the PA wedge pressure, cardiac index and mixed venous oxygen saturation.

The exudation of fluid into the alveolar spaces which is a cardinal feature of ARDS occurs secondary to a low oncotic (osmotic) pressure of the plasma coupled with increased pulmonary capillary permeability. The capillary oncotic pressure is roughly equivalent to 0.57 × serum albumin (grams/litre), and varies between 22–26 mmHg. The difference between this and the wedge pressure is normally about 10 mmHg, but with a falling oncotic pressure, the differential increases and pulmonary oedema will occur despite normal wedge pressures. Monitoring the wedge pressure and oncotic pressure allows fluid balance to be carefully titrated, along with careful oxygenation. Positive end-expiratory pressure ventilation (PEEP) is usually needed to obtain the best oxygen delivery to the tissues, which may be monitored by assessment of the mixed venous oxygen saturation.

Mortality from the ARDS remains high (60–70%), death not always resulting from respiratory failure but more often from multi-organ failure.

Cardiac Output

The cardiac output is the volume of blood ejected from the left ventricle in a period of one minute and is normally between 4–6 litres at rest. In critically ill patients, a reduced cardiac output is usually caused by decreased cardiac contractility. This may be due to ischaemia, to metabolic effects (eg. acidaemia) or to drugs depressing myocardial function (negative inotropic effect). A wide variety of non-cardiac factors may also exist, such as changes in intra-vascular volumes or mean peripheral resistance. Mechanical ventilation, often required for adequate oxygenation of patients requiring intensive care can also have marked effects on the cardiac output. High end-expiratory pressures diminish cardiac output by limiting venous return and directly depressing myocardial contractility. Any coexisting hypo-volaemia will exaggerate this effect. Use of the Swan-Ganz catheter allows monitoring of the changing intra-cardiac pressures and cardiac output as the ventilator is adjusted to optimise oxygenation of the patient.

The cardiac output may be estimated by a technique known as 'thermodilution', first described by Fegler in 1954. Using a modified Swan-Ganz catheter, the change in blood temperature is detected when cold saline is injected into the circulation. The modified Swan-Ganz thermodilution catheter has a right atrial port through which the cold saline may be injected into the circulation, and a thermistor situated near the distal end of the catheter records the temperature change at a point 26 cm farther along in the direction of the blood-stream. The resulting cooling of the blood relates to the cardiac output. In practice, 10 ml of saline or 5% dextrose at 4 °C or room temperature are injected into the right atrium via the 30 cm port. The change in temperature of the blood is recorded by the thermistor at the catheter tip. A bedside computer is used to analyse the heat decay curve which provides a direct read-out of cardiac output. It is usual to take the mean of three consecutive readings to calculate the cardiac output more accurately, and these should not differ by more than 10%. It may also be useful to take the measurements at different phases of the respiratory cycle to allow for the changing cardiac output during inspiration and expiration. Accuracy depends upon smooth injection of the saline bolus and avoiding warming of the fluid before injection. However, if the injection is delivered within 2–4 seconds, the rate of injection does not affect the calculation of cardiac output and automatic injectors are not necessary. The saline should be ice cold (4 °C), and stored in a thermos flask of iced water at the bedside. For additional accuracy, volumes of less than 5 ml should not be used and 10 ml is preferable.

It can be seen that this technique actually measures right ventricular cardiac output, but this is equivalent to the left ventricular output, unless there is an intra-cardiac shunt (due to a septal defect). Left ventricular cardiac output can be measured non-invasively by transthoracic echocardiography.

Continuous Cardiac Output Monitoring

A modified Swan-Ganz catheter is now available which can give a continuous cardiac output reading. A heating element warms the flow of blood in the right atrium in cycles, and the distal thermistor detects the changes between the normal blood temperature and the artificially warmed blood. Such a method has limitations in pyrexial patients but further development may eliminate this drawback.

Cardiac output is often better expressed as cardiac index which relates the output to the size of the patient. It is given by cardiac output (litres/minute) divided by the body surface area (in metres squared). The cardiac index is normally above 2.7 l/min/m^2 (range 2.2 – 4.0), but in the poorly perfused patient will have fallen to 2.0 l/min/m^2. A cardiac index of less than 1.8 l/min/m^2 is typical in patients with cardiogenic shock.

Changes in Cardiac Output

The cardiac output and cardiac index should always be evaluated in the light of clinical appraisal of the patient. Changes in cardiac pre-load, afterload, mean peripheral resistance and contractility may all affect cardiac output.

The cardiac output may either be reduced (as in shock) or increased (as in states of high metabolic demand). Some influences on cardiac output are shown in Table 9.3.

Table 9.3: Some Influences on Cardiac Output

A) Increased Cardiac Output	
Increased metabolic demand:	Septicemia Hyper-thyroidism Anaemia Pregnancy Fevers
Reduced peripheral resistance:	Vasodilator therapy Vasodilator reactions (eg. sepsis)
B) Reduced Cardiac Output	
Reduced venous return (pre-load):	Dehydration Haemorrhage Mechanical ventilation Intra-cardiac shunt (left to right)
Increased after load:	Hypertension Pulmonary embolism Vaso-constriction Cardiac valve stenosis
Depressed cardiac contractility:	Myocardial ischaemia/infarction Drugs (eg. beta-blockers) Acidosis Cardiac tamponade Ventricular aneurysm
Impaired diastolic filling:	Tachycardias Atrial fibrillation
Increased pre-load*:	Fluid overload Incompetent valves Intra-cardiac shunt (right to left)
Inappropriate heart rate:	Bradycardias Tachycardias

* When the myocardium is over-stretched, and Starling's Law is exceeded

Indications for Pulmonary Artery Wedge Pressure Monitoring

Generally, the Swan-Ganz catheter is employed where cardio-pulmonary pressures, blood flow and circulating volumes require precise and intensive management. The anticipated benefits however must outweigh the risks and expense of the procedure.

There are essentially two main indications for the measurement of the wedge pressure: low output states and pulmonary oedema. In both cases, haemodynamic monitoring with a pulmonary artery catheter can provide clinical data which might be useful both diagnostically and therapeutically.

a) Low output states

Significant reductions in cardiac output are usually either due to left ventricular (pump) failure or hypo-volaemia. However, in critically ill patients these two factors may coexist and distinction may be difficult. The presence of a raised jugular venous pressure and peripheral oedema do not exclude hypo-volaemia, and may occur in conditions such as right ventricular myocardial infarction, chronic obstructive airways disease, pulmonary embolism and right-sided valvular disease. If the patient is hypo-volaemic, arterial blood pressure is initially maintained by an increase in the mean peripheral resistance and a tachycardia which compensates for the reduction in cardiac output. Eventually, left ventricular filling pressures will fall and the cardiac output will decline, often critically. This is recognisable immediately if serial wedge pressures and/or cardiac output measurements are being recorded. If the development of shock is not due to hypo-volaemia, but due to left ventricular (pump) failure, there is a fall in cardiac output but a rise in the wedge pressure, since the heart cannot eject the volume load. Here the wedge pressure is giving an indication of left ventricular performance. In both these cases, assessment of the CVP alone will only be of value if right ventricular failure has occurred secondary to failure of the left ventricle. Measurement of the wedge pressure will of course allow recognition of left ventricular failure before it extends to the right ventricle.

Pulmonary embolism may also produce a confusing haemodynamic picture, especially if it complicates acute myocardial infarction. A raised PA pressure with a normal or low left atrial (PAWP) pressure will allow the aetiology of induced hypotension to be correctly diagnosed as embolic rather than left ventricular failure.

Data obtained by the Swan-Ganz catheter has also been used to determine prognosis in patients following acute myocardial infarction by measurement of the cardiac index and wedge pressure (Table 9.4). This data allows selection of the most appropriate treatment.

Table 9.4: Classification, Therapy and Mortality if Patients following acute myocardial infarction

Class	Cardiac Output	Index*	Wedge Pressure (mmHg)	Therapy	Mortality (%)
No cardiac failure	Normal	>2.2	<18	Bed rest	3
Pulmonary congestion	Normal	>2.2	>18	Lower wedge pressure with: diuretics (blood pressure normal) vasodilators (blood pressure raised)	9
Peripheral hypo-perfusion	Low	<2.2	<18	Plasma expanders	23
Pulmonary congestion and peripheral hypo-perfusion	Low	<2.2	>18	Reduce wedge pressure with diuretics/ vasodilators If hypotensive, use inotropic agents	51

*Cardiac index (1/min per m^2) = cardiac output (litres) per minute per body surface area (m^2) (From Forrester et al., 1976. Reproduced by kind permission of the *New England Journal of Medicine*)

b) Pulmonary oedema

Pulmonary oedema may occur secondary to increased pulmonary permeability, increased hydrostatic pressure, decreased plasma oncotic pressure or perhaps all three together. Determining the underlying pathological mechanism which produces the classical appearance of pulmonary oedema on the chest X-ray is a familiar clinical dilemma. Most cases will be due to raised hydrostatic pressure (as occurs in left ventricular failure), or increased capillary permeability (as occurs in the respiratory distress syndrome). These can be distinguished by measurement of wedge pressure, since low or normal pressures are found in the latter case, and high pressures in the former.

It is also worth remembering that it may take up to 48 hours following haemodynamic stabilisation for the resolution of abnormal physical and radiological signs.

The whole range of data obtained by the Swan-Ganz catheter may be processed by programmable computers to calculate other parameters which cannot be directly measured, including stroke volume, stroke work, systemic and pulmonary vascular resistance.

Problems with Pulmonary Artery Monitoring

Although passage of the Swan-Ganz catheter is usually easy, measurement of the wedge pressure meets with difficulty in 25–30% of cases. It is obviously important that the data obtained is correct; there are four criteria that may be employed to validate the accuracy of the wedge pressure reading:

1) Firstly, the wedge pressure must be less than the PA pressure. Artifactual elevation of the wedge pressure may be produced by 'over-wedging', when the balloon is inflated eccentrically, such that the tip is pushed against the vessel wall, or when the distal lumen is partially occluded by the balloon herniating over the tip. Wedge pressure estimation is particularly difficult in patients with pulmonary hypertension. Sufficient time should be allowed for the pressures to settle following balloon inflation.

2) The wedge tracing must be consistent with the left atrial (venous) pressure waveform, resembling the classical *a*, *c* and *v* waves.

3) Free flow of the infusion solution should be possible in the wedge position which indicates that the tip is not occluded.

4) The blood PO_2 during wedge sampling should not be greater than in a non-wedge sample.

Complications

Complications arising from the use of Swan-Ganz catheters are infrequent, but careful observation of the patient before during and up to 24 hours following withdrawal of the catheter is desirable. The more frequent problems include:

a) Dysrhythmias

Rhythm disturbances during catheter insertion include heart block, atrial and ventricular tachycardias. The frequency of dysrhythmias is much higher in those with predisposing conditions including hypoxia, acute myocardial infarction and electrolyte imbalance. Dysrhythmias are caused by mechanical irritation of the endocardium or valves, and are usually noted at the time of catheter insertion, manipulation or removal. Occasionally, they may be caused by catheter knotting or the catheter tip falling back into the right ventricle. Continuous ECG monitoring is desirable especially during catheter operation. Resuscitation facilities must also be available.

b) Infection

Infection is a common complication with all centrally placed lines. There are many reasons for this including breaks in the closed system for blood sampling or injection of fluid boluses for cardiac output calculation. Repeated catheter manipulation may also produce an inflammatory response, as may migration of unsterile portions of the catheter into the veins. Critically ill patients are at increased risk of infection because of decreased immunological status, and prophylactic antibiotic therapy may be required, especially if there is known cardiac valve disease.

Infection may be localised to the insertion site, and is often preceded by thrombophlebitis which is caused by mechanical irritation of the vein, and is more common when the ante-cubital fossa is being used for access. Movement of the catheter may be minimised if it is fixed to the skin with sutures and then looped under the dressing to prevent direct traction. Use of the ante-cubital vein is not preferred because of the long length of cannula in contact with the vein. If this approach is used, the arm should be immobilised with an arm board. The insertion site should be observed daily for redness, swelling and drainage. This may be made easier if a see-through dressing is employed. The dressing may then remain undisturbed, provided there are no signs of infection. With the traditional gauze dressing, inspection is required within 48 hours of insertion, and then every 24 hours. Application of an antibiotic cream may inhibit bacterial growth. After catheter removal, the catheter tip and an insertion site swab should be sent for culture. The site should be cleaned, antibiotic cream applied and a dry dressing placed over the wound. Any sutures may be removed at 72 hours.

A catheter-related septicaemia is an uncommon but serious complication. It may be the explanation for a pyrexia of unknown origin. The catheter must be removed immediately. Blood cultures should be taken via the monitoring lumen prior to catheter removal and the tip of the catheter sent for culture. Endocarditis may follow.

As with all centrally placed lines, scrupulous asepsis is required before, during and after catheter insertion, especially during catheter manipulation or during injections of fluids. If the catheter is not secured to the skin, then migration of the unsterile portion may occur. A permanent indwelling introducer and polythene sleeve may be used to protect the proximal 30 cm of the catheter, and allow catheter manipulation without compromising sterility (Figure 9.3).

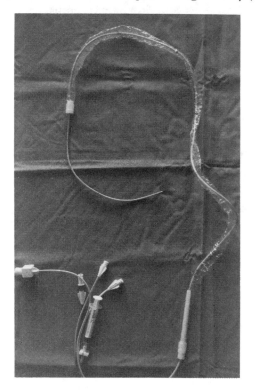

Figure 9.3 Polythene sleeve protector

c) Pulmonary infarction

Pulmonary infarction may result from prolonged, frequent or over-inflation of the balloon, or by thrombus formation around the catheter tip. Patients with a low cardiac output and increased blood coagulability are at particular risk. A continuous flushing system should be utilised with heparin to minimise thrombus formation. After blood sampling, the system should be fast-flushed to clear the line. Any obvious clot should be removed by aspiration. During recording the PAWP, the balloon should not be inflated for more than 15 seconds and then deflated immediately. Another cause of pulmonary infarction is due to catheter migration which occurs spontaneously over a period of time. The catheter tip then wedges in a pulmonary capillary, causing obstruction. To prevent this, the catheter tip should be pulled well back into the pulmonary artery after wedge pressure measurement, and if the insertion cannula has a retention screw, this should be tightened. Continuous display of the pressure waveform will also immediately demonstrate if the catheter tip has moved into the wedge position. Pressure damping caused by thrombus formation should also be visible.

d) Perforation of the pulmonary artery

If the balloon is inflated too quickly, it may rupture or cause rupture of a pulmonary capillary. The latter is rare, although patients with long-standing pulmonary disease are at risk. Balloon inflation should always be slow and must only be done whilst watching the pressure trace for signs of wedging before the balloon is fully inflated. Pulling the tip well back into the pulmonary artery after recording the wedge should prevent this. The catheter should not be advanced with the balloon deflated.

e) Balloon rupture and air embolism

Balloon rupture becomes more likely if the catheter has been left in place for prolonged periods or if it is inflated too many times. The thin latex balloon absorbs lipoproteins from the blood and gradually loses its elasticity. Few balloons can withstand more than 70 inflations, and the catheter probably does not last beyond 72 hours.

Balloon rupture should be suspected when there is no resistance to attempted inflation, and there is failure to wedge. It is probably not harmful to release 1.5 ml of air into the pulmonary circulation, but if there is a right-to-left shunt in the heart (for example, through a septal defect) peripheral air embolisation may result, and use of carbon dioxide to inflate the catheter balloon is preferable in the at-risk patient. The Swan-Ganz catheter comes with its own fixed-volume syringe which should be used to prevent over inflation of the balloon and releasing too much air into the circulation if the balloon ruptures.

f) Catheter kinking and intra-cardiac knotting

This rare complication may be caused if excessive lengths of the catheter are inserted. The right atrium is about 35 cm from the neck veins and the pulmonary artery 15 cm beyond. The ante-cubital route adds about 35 cm to these figures. Catheter length inserted may be checked against the black markings on the catheter. If knotting or kinking occurs, slow withdrawal is usually all that is required.

Chapter 10
Monitoring Blood Gases and Acid–Base Balance

Respiratory function has to adapt to many changing circumstances to control the arterial blood gases in health and disease. The pulmonary blood flow is about 5 litres per minute, which carries 250 ml of oxygen to the tissues. At the same time, normal respiration removes 200 ml of carbon dioxide from the body. The arterial gas tensions (pressures) are closely controlled to keep oxygen (PaO_2) at 80–100 mmHg (10.7–13.3 kPa) and carbon dioxide ($PaCO_2$) at 35–45 mmHg (4.7–6.0 kPa) whilst air is being breathed.

Although the pulmonary circulation receives the same amount of blood as the systemic circulation (the cardiac output is identical through each side of the heart), the pulmonary vascular resistance is only one-sixth of the peripheral resistance. This is because the pulmonary vascular bed is very distensible, and pulmonary capillaries can open and close in response to changing haemodynamic pressures. If the systemic resistance rises, the pulmonary resistance falls.

Alveolar Ventilation and Perfusion

Maximal efficiency of oxygenation requires matching of alveolar ventilation (termed 'V') and alveolar perfusion (termed 'Q'). A mismatch of ventilation and perfusion (*V/Q mismatch*) is obviously inefficient. There is no point in perfusing an alveolus if it is not being ventilated, and vice versa. Two mechanisms operate to match ventilation and perfusion.

a) A low PO_2 produces local vaso-constriction which 'shunts' blood away from the underventilated area.

b)   A reduced $PaCO_2$ (perhaps caused by a vessel being blocked by thrombus) causes local bronchiole constriction, so that ventilation to the region is reduced.

In a normal adult, about 5% of the blood passing from the lungs is deoxygenated because of physiological shunting, but during respiratory tract infections, areas of the lung may collapse thus, increasing the shunt.

The concentration of oxygen in air is about 21%, but in medical practice inspired air is commonly enriched with supplemental oxygen delivered by oxygen masks or ventilators if there is impairment or failure of respiration. The oxygen concentration is often expressed as a fraction (0.21) called the *fractional oxygen concentration (FIO₂)* of inspired gas. Raising the FIO_2 will help to correct hypoxaemia, reduce the work of breathing and decrease myocardial work.

Respiratory failure describes the failure to oxygenate the blood appropriately, or remove carbon dioxide sufficiently and may be defined as a PaO_2 below 60 mmHg (8 kPa), which may occur with or without a rise in the $PaCO_2$ (Table 10.1).

Whilst significant carbon dioxide retention is associated with warm vaso-dilated peripheries, headaches, tachycardia, flapping tremor and confusion, mild to moderate hypoxaemia is a common,

Table 10.1: Definition of Respiratory Failure

Type 1 Respiratory Failure

PaO_2 < 60 mmHg (< 8 kPa)
$PaCO_2$ < 45 mmHg (< 6.5 kPa)

This form of respiratory failure results from a mismatch of ventilation and perfusion or diffusion in the lungs

Examples:
Pneumonia, left ventricular failure, fibrosing alveolitis, adult respiratory distress syndrome, pulmonary emboli

Type 2 Respiratory Failure

PaO_2 < 60 mmHg (< 8 kPa)
$PaCO_2$ > 45 mmHg (> 6.5 kPa)

This indicates that alveolar ventilation is inadequate for metabolic needs, and is sometimes referred to as 'ventilatory failure'. It may occur with or without ventilation/perfusion mismatching

Examples:
Chronic bronchitis, chest injuries or deformity, drugs depressing the respiratory centre (eg. opiates)

---

often asymptomatic disorder which may be found in many patients. The most frequent and important cause of hypoxaemia is produced by a ventilation/perfusion mismatch where areas of the lung which are poorly oxygenated compared to their arterial perfusion (eg. pneumonia), or where parts of the lung are ventilated normally, but the blood perfusion is inadequate (eg. pulmonary embolism).

Hypoxaemia is often poorly detected by clinical means unless it is severe enough to produce cyanosis. An accurate determination of the arterial blood gases and oxygen saturation is often required for formulating the correct diagnosis and subsequently monitoring the critically ill patient.

Whilst oximetric assessment of arterial oxygen saturation (SaO_2) is now easily acquired non-invasively at the bedside, full blood gas analysis is required to provide information about arterial oxygen and carbon dioxide tensions (PaO_2 and $PaCO_2$), pH, bicarbonate (HCO_3) and base excess (BE), the latter three being important for understanding the patient's acid–base balance. Blood gas analysis is, however, more difficult, requiring arterial puncture and the avail-ability of an automated blood gas analyser. The normal values for blood gases and associated parameters are shown in Table 10.2.

Table 10.2: Normal Blood Gas Values and Other Associated Parameters

	Arterial blood	Mixed venous blood
pH	7.35–7.45	7.33–7.43
PaO_2	80–100 mmHg (10.7–13.3 kPa)	37–42 mmHg (5–5.6kPa)
$PaCO_2$	35–45 mmHg (4.7–6.0 kPa)	42–50 mmHg (5.6–6.7 kPa)
HCO_3	22–26 mmol/l	24–28 mmol/l
BE	–2 – +2 mmol/l	0–4 mmol/l
SaO_2	95% or greater	65–80%

Older people tend to have PaO_2 and SaO_2 levels nearer the lower end of the ranges, whereas younger patients tend to have higher normal values. Mixed venous blood gas tensions are more variable.

Arterial Blood Gas Sampling

The reliability of arterial blood gas analysis depends both upon the correct sampling technique and the proper handling of the sample. The common sites for obtaining arterial blood are the radial artery at the wrist and the femoral artery in the groin, but the brachial artery of the non-dominant arm is probably the site of choice (just above the elbow). It is preferable to select a glass syringe or a plastic syringe with a vented plunger to take the sample. Both will allow the syringe to fill without manually pulling on the plunger. If a normal syringe is chosen, the plunger has to be physically withdrawn which makes it impossible to be sure that the blood sample is arterial rather than venous in origin. About 1 ml of heparin (1000 units/ml) should be drawn into the syringe, and allowed to wet the barrel before being expelled. The dead-space in the syringe hub will then contain enough heparin to adequately anti-coagulate the blood as the sample is taken. Excess amounts of heparin should be avoided since it may cause haemolysis and the falsely reduce the pH of the specimen. The course of the brachial artery is defined by placing the middle and index fingers along the line of maximal pulsation, and then the needle is advanced slowly between them and into the artery. Arterial blood should enter the syringe easily, with pulsation. It will not necessarily be bright red. A 'butterfly' type needle is sometimes used for arterial puncture, which allows the blood to pulsate up the tubing. However, this may allow oxygenation of the sample by the air, and the first part of the specimen will need to be discarded. Specimens which include air bubbles will give falsely elevated oxygen results; bubbles should be expelled at once, and the nozzle end of the syringe sealed. The sample should be mixed gently to ensure adequate anti-coagulation and then be placed on ice to prevent red cell metabolism occurring during transport to the laboratory. Delays in analysis will allow metabolic changes which will reduce the PaO_2 and alter the pH. The most common concern is accidental venous sampling. It is not possible to determine from the results alone whether or not this was the case, particularly when dealing with critically ill patients who may be acidotic and cyanosed. If venous sampling is suspected, a known venous sample should be taken for blood gas analysis and the two results compared. If the results are similar, the first sample was venous, but if the PaO_2 and SaO_2 are significantly lower, then a true arterial sample was taken initially.

Firm pressure must be applied to the arterial puncture site for at least 5 minutes after sampling, and longer if the patient has been taking anti-coagulants, to prevent haematoma formation.

What is Measured

Modern blood gas analysers use micro-electrodes and may require only 0.2 ml of heparinised blood to make the analysis. The following results are normally provided within 2–3 minutes:

a) Arterial oxygen tension (PaO_2)

The PaO_2 is the partial pressure (tension) of oxygen in arterial blood and is an indicator of the adequacy of oxygenation of the blood by the lungs. The normal range for the PaO_2 in an adult patient breathing room air is shown in Table 10.2. Oxygen therapy is usually required in the adult patient when the PaO_2 is less than 60 mmHg. Severe hypoxaemia (PaO_2 < 30 mmHg) is associated with imminent death. Hypoxaemia is usually due to a ventilation/perfusion mismatch in the lungs, although it may be due to hypo-ventilation or right to left cardiac shunts. Hypoxia due to impaired oxygen diffusion across the alveolar wall usually only occurs during exercise, but may be a feature of the respiratory distress syndrome.

b) Arterial carbon dioxide tension (PaCO₂)

The concentration of carbonic acid in the plasma is determined by the partial pressure (tension) of carbon dioxide in the alveoli (PCO_2). This is maintained by balancing the rate of carbon dioxide production (by the tissues), and the respiratory rate (which removes carbon dioxide from the body). The $PaCO_2$ is therefore an indicator of the efficiency of ventilation, and normally lies between 35–45 mmHg. A $PaCO_2$ greater than 45 mmHg therefore indicates hypo-ventilation (CO_2 is retained), whereas a $PaCO_2$ less than 35 mmHg indicates hyper-ventilation (CO_2 is 'blown off').

c) pH

The blood is normally alkaline because it contains bicarbonate, phosphate and proteins which are strong bases. These are partially balanced by carbonic acid. The degree of acidity or alkalinity of the blood is measured using either direct measurement of the hydrogen ion content (normally 35–45 nmol/l), or more usually by using a logarithmic expression of the hydrogen ion concentration called the pH (normal range 7.35 –7.45). During normal metabolism, the body produces large amounts of acid, which may be excreted through the kidneys or via the lung (as carbon dioxide). In addition, the blood is able to buffer fluctuations so that the blood pH is kept within narrow limits to assure optimal cellular function. If these mechanisms break down, then the patient will become acidotic (pH less than 7.35) or alkalotic (pH greater than 7.45).

d) Standard bicarbonate (HCO₃⁻)

Bicarbonate is one of the body's main bases and represents the renal regulated, metabolic component of the acid–base balance. When reported in a blood gas sample, the plasma bicarbonate concentration is expressed as a calculated value equilibrated at a PCO_2 of 40 mmHg/5.3 kPa (the usual PCO_2 in the alveoli). This avoids artificial elevation of the plasma bicarbonate at high $PaCO_2$ levels. An HCO_3 less than 22 mmol/l indicates a metabolic acidoses, whereas a value greater than 26 mmol/l indicates a metabolic alkalosis or bicarbonate excess.

e) Base excess

Base excess is a reflection of the total non-respiratory acid–base balance, and represents the buffering capacity of the blood. It is automatically calculated at a PCO_2 of 40 mmHg/5.3 kPa so that only the metabolic (rather than the respiratory) component of excess acidity or alkalinity is given. The range is –2 to +2 mmol/l. If positive, the sample is alkaline, if negative, the sample is acidic.

Acid–Base Balance

There are four common metabolic disturbances which may be described briefly as:

1) Metabolic acidosis

A metabolic acidosis results from accumulation of acids such as occurs in diabetic keto-acidosis, lactic acidosis or aspirin overdose. In renal failure it is due to accumulation of creatinine, sulphates and phosphates. Hydrogen ions (H^+) are 'mopped up' by bicarbonate (HCO_3^-), producing more carbon dioxide which is then blown off. The primary biochemical effect is a fall in the bicarbonate concentration followed clinically by hyperventilation to remove the carbon dioxide. A metabolic acidosis may also result from bicarbonate loss, as may occur in profuse diarrhoea or leakage of pancreatic juices.

2) Metabolic alkalosis

This may result from profuse vomiting, when acid is lost, leaving an excess of bicarbonate ions. Long-term Ryles tube aspiration will have the same effect. Rarely it may complicate steroid therapy, or may be seen in severe potassium depletion.

The pH, the base excess and the bicarbonate levels are raised.

3) Respiratory alkalosis

Hyperventilation causes increased carbon dioxide excretion (resulting in a low $PaCO_2$), with consequent hydrogen ion loss and rise in the pH. The bicarbonate concentration tends to remain constant unless the situation is chronic.

The reasons for hyperventilation may include hysteria, hypoxia, cardiac failure, pulmonary embolism, asthma or anaemia.

4) Respiratory acidosis

This implies a high $PaCO_2$ due to hypoventilation resulting from obstructive pulmonary disease, depression of the respiratory centre (drugs, or raised intracranial pressure) or some neuromuscular disorders. With increasing hydrogen ion production the pH falls.

Ventilation and Acid–Base Balance

There is a tight inverse relationship between the blood pH and ventilation. Clinically, this is apparent by the deep and rapid (Kussmaul) respiration observed in acute renal failure or diabetic keto-acidosis. The increase in respiratory rate enables the soluble carbon dioxide to be 'blown off' by the lungs to return the pH to normal. This is termed respiratory compensation for a metabolic acidosis.

Conversely, when there is carbon dioxide retention (eg. chronic obstructive airways disease), there is a metabolic compensation for this respiratory acidosis by bicarbonate retention with excretion of acid urine to keep the blood pH normal.

Other Methods of Assessing Oxygenation

The use of arterial blood gas sampling is limited because it is invasive and only provides an intermittent estimation of the blood gases and acid–base status. Additionally, because the analysers are often sited away from the bedside, there are sometimes delays in the transmission of results to the clinician. Alternatives for assessing adequacy of oxygenation such as oximetry and transcutaneous blood gas monitoring have therefore been developed to enable continuous, non-invasive assessment of the blood gases.

A: Pulse Oximetry

Pulse oximetry assesses arterial blood oxygen saturation using a probe which is usually placed on the finger or ear (Figure 10.1). Oximeters can also be mounted on modified pulmonary artery catheters to extend the role of Swan-Ganz monitoring when invasive studies are being carried out (see Chapter 9).

Blood Oxygen Content and Haemoglobin Saturation

Haemoglobin is responsible for carrying most of the oxygen in the blood (97%), each gram combining with approximately 1.38 ml of

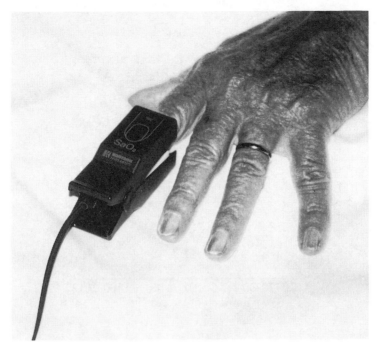

Figure 10.1 Oximeter finger probe

oxygen. The remaining 3% of the circulating oxygen is dissolved in the plasma. The total of amount of oxygen carried is known as the *oxygen content* and is equivalent to about 19.7 ml of oxygen per 100 ml of blood.

The *oxygen saturation* (SaO_2) reflects how much of this oxygen carrying capacity by the haemoglobin is being utilised. Thus:

$$\text{Oxygen saturation } (SaO_2) = \frac{\text{Amount of oxygen being carried by the haemoglobin}}{\text{Amount that can be carried by the haemoglobin}}$$

When haemoglobin carries oxygen, it is converted to oxy-haemoglobin, and the amount of oxygen which is able to be carried is closely related to the PO_2 of the blood, the relationship being shown in the oxy-haemoglobin dissociation curve (Figure 10.2). This shows that the correlation between the PO_2 and oxygen saturation is not linear, but 'S' shaped. This relationship shows that in parts of the body where the PO_2 is low (eg. in the peripheral capillary beds) saturation is low, the oxygen having passed into the tissues. In areas where the PO_2 is high (eg. the lungs), the haemoglobin is able to combine with, and carry much more oxygen and is therefore highly saturated.

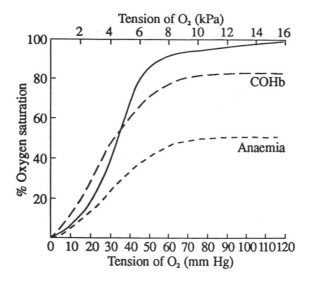

Figure 10.2 The oxy-haemoglobin dissociation curve. The effects of anaemia and heavy smoking on oxygen carriage are shown. Smokers have high levels of circulating carboxy-haemoglobin (COHb).

When assessing the need for oxygen therapy, it is important to remember that it is the oxygen content and saturation of the blood which is more important than the arterial oxygen tension. Hypoxaemia is present if either the PaO_2 or the content of oxygen in arterial blood is reduced. For example, in anaemia, all the blood may be saturated, but the oxygen content will be low.

The arterial oxygen content may be calculated by multiplying 1.38 (the amount of oxygen carried by one gram of haemoglobin), by the haemoglobin concentration (g/dl), by the oxygen saturation (SaO_2 percentage).

Hence, for a haemoglobin of 15 g/dl which is 95% saturated, the oxygen content will be:

$$1.38 \times 15 \times 95 = 19.7 \text{ ml per 100 ml blood}$$

Indications for Pulse Oximetry

Oximetry is widely utilised in primary care and hospital practice (Table 10.3). Despite some limitations, it has become one of the most important advances in patient monitoring techniques.

Continuous monitoring with pulse oximetry has become routine in anaesthetic practice, and is increasingly found in other acute care areas such as endoscopy units and cardiac care units. Because it is so easy to perform and may give additional data during the assessment of acutely ill patients, the technique is likely to become more widespread.

Table 10.3: Some Clinical Uses of Pulse Oximetry

Coronary and Intensive Care Units – during routine cardiovascular monitoring

During and after anaesthesia – to evaluate hypoxaemia peri-operatively and in the recovery room

Endoscopy Units – during bronchoscopy and gastroscopy when breathing may be compromised

Accident and Emergency Units – in evaluating patients who have chronic pulmonary disease, those who are restless and confused (possibly due to hypoxia) or have chest injuries

Whilst arterial puncture is necessary if the $PaCO_2$ or acid–base state is being assessed, many patients have arterial samples taken solely to assess the PaO_2. If an estimation of oxygenation is all that is needed, pulse oximetry is usually sufficient. In addition, since correct technique and attention to detail are often lacking in those who only occasionally perform arterial puncture, the blood gas results may be subject to error (the PaO_2 is usually overestimated), and there may be a risk of harm to the patient. Since pulse oximetry is non-invasive and less prone to user error, it gives a more accurate estimation of oxygenation in the majority of cases.

How it Works

The principle of oximetry was developed following the simple observation that oxygenated and deoxygenated blood differ in colour; arterial blood appears red while venous blood appears blue. When the two are mixed, the ratio of their concentrations can be determined from the amount of light absorbed at two different wavelengths. Oximetry uses this principle to measure the ratio of the concentrations of oxygenated to the total concentration in arterial blood in pulsatile capillaries by the amount of red and infra-red light absorbed. A detector calculates this ratio as these light sources shine through the capillary beds in the extremities (usually the finger tip, or ear) and expresses the result as a percentage.

The oximeter probe contains the two light emitting diodes (one red and one infra-red) which shine towards a detector located opposite (Figure 10.3). The diodes are rapidly switched on and off, and the detector records how much of the light has been absorbed on its passage through the tissues. The oximeter makes an allowance for the amount of light in the room or, more specifically, shining on the detector. The latter estimation is important since excessive ambient light (for example, from operating theatre lights) may saturate the detector and produce inaccurate readings. After making corrections for this ambient light, the ratio of red to infra-red light is determined. In order to eliminate the light-absorbing effects of other tissues, the resulting signal registers only the readings from blood pulsating in the capillaries (hence 'pulsed' oximetry). The corresponding arterial oxygen saturation is calculated as an average based on the previous few seconds of recording which is constantly being updated. The results are displayed as the percentage oxy-haemoglobin saturation.

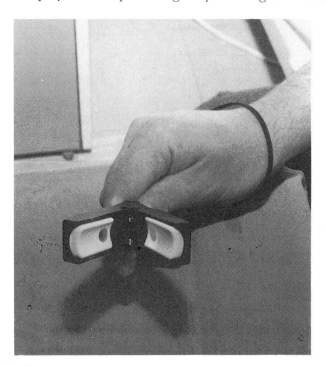

Figure 10.3 Close up of oximeter probe

The relationship between oxygen saturation and oxygen tension is depicted in the oxy-haemoglobin dissociation curve (see Figure 10.2). It can be seen that target arterial oxygen saturation should be viewed as at least 90% which equates with the end of the plateau after which saturation falls quite rapidly as the PaO_2 declines. Oxygen therapy should be given to raise the SaO_2 to at least 90%. If the SaO$_2$ is found to be less than 80%, arterial blood gases should additionally be taken to obtain a complete picture.

This target saturation will vary since the oxygen dissociation curve shifts when carbon dioxide, pH and body temperature are altered. Acidaemia, carbon dioxide retention and pyrexia will all push the curve to the right ('right shift') causing decreased affinity of the blood for oxygen. This means that although less oxygen is picked up in the lungs, it is more readily delivered to the tissues. Hyperventilation, alkalosis and hypo-thermia shifts the curve to the left ('left shift'). In this situation, the blood oxygen content for any given PaO$_2$ is higher. More oxygen is picked up in the lungs, but less is delivered to the tissues. Thus, evaluation of the patient's arterial oxygen saturation needs these variables to be considered.

Problems with Monitoring

The following factors may lead to poor recording of the arterial saturation during pulse oximetry:

a) Poor tissue perfusion

The pulse oximeter can only function if enough pulsatile blood passes between the light source and the detector. If tissue perfusion is poor or the pulse is weak, the generated signal will be liable to error. Poor perfusion may be indicated by an automatic warning message from the instrument itself or may be deduced by observing the shape of the arterial pulse waveform. If perfusion is good, there is a sharp arterial waveform, often with a clear dicrotic notch (see Figure 8.3 page 129). If perfusion is poor, the arterial waveform is abnormal. In this case, the accuracy of the displayed saturation value should be viewed with caution, and an attempt should be made to either improve perfusion at the chosen site or to move the probe to a different site.

b) Abnormal haemoglobins

Compounds that absorb light at the same wavelengths as haemoglobin and oxy-haemoglobin will introduce errors (eg. nail varnish!). The microprocessor in the oximeter is programmed to parameters derived from the normal oxyhemoglobin dissociation curve. Hence, such problems as abnormal haemoglobins (foetal haemoglobin, carboxy- and met-haemoglobin) may produce errors. In most of these cases, the oximeter will underestimate the true saturation, and mislead the clinician into thinking that there is a problem, where there is not. Of far more concern is situations where the oximeter may over-estimate saturation. The most common is with carboxy-haemoglobin, which leads to an overestimation of the true concentration of oxy-haemoglobin.

Carboxy-haemoglobin may form 5–10% of the total haemoglobin in heavy smokers, and even higher concentrations in those admitted to hospital following inhalation of carbon monoxide. Arterial oxygen saturation will be high, but it will not be delivered to the tissues. Carboxy-haemoglobin has an affinity for oxygen 300 times that of haemoglobin; oxygen will bind preferentially with it and not be released in the capillary beds.

c) Excessive ambient light

Excessive ambient light may saturate the detector and cause erroneous readings. This is particularly so if there is strong sunlight shining on the probe, or flickering fluorescent lights. Ambient light is a particular problem if the finger is not fully inserted into a finger probe, allowing external light sources to fall on the detector. A lopsided probe will allow light from the two light emitters to pass directly into the detector, and not through the tissues of the finger.

d) Motion artifact

Most motion artifact occurs from the probe slipping across the skin whenever the hand is moved. The probe and cable should be adequately secured to the patient. The cable should be long enough to permit the patient to move, and it is sometimes useful to fix a 'stress loop' in the cable to the skin, so that traction does not occur directly on the probe. Whilst clip-type probes attached to the fingers are suitable in most cases, self-adhesive probes should be substituted if long-term monitoring is intended. Care is required with children who may be burned if these probes are stuck in one place for too long. Using the toes is sometimes possible, but poor perfusion at this site is more likely to make readings unreliable. Persistent limb tremor is an occasional problem best circumvented by application of the ear probe. The probe is clipped to the ear lobe or pinna, ensuring that the clip does not pinch the skin and thus impair perfusion.

B: Transcutaneous Blood Gas Monitoring

Oxygen and carbon dioxide are able to diffuse through the skin if perfusion is good enough, and can be detected by means of electro-chemical sensors applied to the skin surface. Transcutaneous blood gas monitoring can therefore provide another non-invasive way of monitoring blood gases continuously.

Transcutaneous oxygen monitoring measures the PO_2 at tissue level ($PtcO_2$), which is dependent both on the PaO_2 and tissue perfusion. When perfusion is normal, $PtcO_2$ correlates well with the PaO_2, although in patients with a low cardiac output or tissue oedema, perfusion is poor, tissue delivery of oxygen is impaired and under these conditions the $PtcO_2$ will be low despite a normal PaO_2.

There is a usually a good correlation between the $PtcO_2$ and PaO_2 in infants, but the thicker skin of adults may make this correlation less reliable. In addition, for this technique to work the skin has to be heated to about 44 °C to allow oxygen diffusion and accidental burning may occur.

The machinery is cumbersome and expensive with a tendency to overestimate hypoxia, so the technique has mostly been superseded by pulse oximetry. However, since transcutaneous monitoring gives a more consistent picture of tissue oxygenation than arterial blood gases do, the technique is probably better at indicating the viability of ischaemic limbs and tissue flaps which are clinical situations where pulse oximetry is not valid.

Monitoring Mixed Venous Oxygen Saturation

Although assessment of the cardiac output gives a good guide to the circulatory status, it does not necessarily indicate the adequacy of oxygen delivery to the tissues. Since the ultimate goal of treating hypoxia is adequate tissue oxygenation, a more sensitive guide for the adjustment of oxygen therapy may be monitoring the mixed venous oxygen saturation (SVO_2). A suitable sample of mixed venous blood may be obtained from the tip of a pulmonary artery catheter. This blood which has travelled all around the body, has been mixed in the heart, and is just about to be re-oxygenated. Sampling from the CVP line is not as good; if it lies in the superior vena cava, it will only represent venous blood returning from the head and neck, and if in the right atrium, not enough time may have elapsed for efficient mixing before sampling.

Whilst intermittent aspiration of mixed venous blood is usual practice, continuous monitoring is now possible using a fibre-optic pulmonary artery catheter. This modified four-channel pulmonary artery catheter has two fibre-optic channels running the whole length of the catheter. Light is emitted down one channel and reflected up the other. Using two light sources at different wavelengths, the electronics are able to calculate the ratio of haemoglobin to oxy-haemoglobin, and hence calculate mixed venous oxygen saturation which is displayed as a continuous numeric display.

The mixed venous oxygen saturation reflects oxygen utilisation by the body tissues, and may be used to assess tissue metabolism. The normal SVO_2 lies between 70–80%, and values in this order infer that the tissues are receiving enough oxygen, and thus that cardio-respiratory function is normal. The SVO_2 will be decreased where there is:

a)   Low arterial oxygen saturation in the pulmonary circulation due to poor oxygenation of the blood by abnormal lungs

b)   Normal arterial saturation in the pulmonary circulation, but a decreased cardiac output slows peripheral blood flow and allows more oxygen extraction in the tissues

c)   A combination of (a) and (b).

If it is known that the PaO_2 is normal (indicating normal lung function), then a low SVO_2 implies that the circulation is failing.

A high SVO_2 is found in sepsis with peripheral shunting or hypothermia.

Monitoring the arterial and mixed venous oxygen saturation together helps to define the relationship between oxygen supply and demand. This information helps determine the best mode of respiratory support, and aids decisions on strategies to improve oxygen transport and reduce oxygen demands.

Monitoring Oxygen Therapy

As oxygen is a drug, it should be prescribed rather than used as a placebo as is commonly witnessed on many hospital wards. The prescription should be in writing, with the intended oxygen concentration (FIO_2) indicated clearly. Oxygen therapy should always be continuous rather than intermittent.

Correct utilisation of oxygen therapy requires:

a)   Ensuring appropriate use of oxygen
b)   Ensuring the correct fractional inspired oxygen concentration
c)   Ensuring adequate humidification
d)   Ensuring proper use by the patient
e)   Preventing carbon dioxide retention.

a) Appropriate use of oxygen

Oxygen should be used as a temporary measure to correct hypoxia, whilst the underlying problem is treated and should be given continuously. Intermittent use of oxygen may be harmful, particularly in severely hypoxic patients, where intermittent therapy may lead to rebound hypoxia. The success of treatment must be based upon frequent estimations of oxygen saturation and/or arterial blood gases. The aim is usually to raise the PaO_2 to at least 60 mmHg (8 kPa), with higher targets being used in patients with a low cardiac output, or where there is local ischaemia.

b) Control over the fraction of inspired oxygen (FIO2)

Inspired air may be supplemented with oxygen delivered either by oxygen masks or by mechanical ventilators. Supplemental oxygen is also usually required for most patients requiring critical care with or without primary pulmonary pathology. Many patients have abnormal lung function due to poor pulmonary perfusion, shunting or ventilation/perfusion mismatches.

Oxygen masks

Oxygen masks are designed to permit either slight oxygen enrichment of the inspired air without re-breathing expired carbon dioxide, or produce high concentrations of oxygen in the inspired air. Lower concentrations of oxygen are usually delivered by semi-open oro-nasal masks working by the Venturi principle (Ventimasks, Vickers Medical Group), and will deliver 24%, 28% or 35% oxygen depending on the oxygen flow rate. Modifications of the Ventimask (Venticaire) are designed to function at flow rates between 2–15 litres/minute and will deliver higher concentrations of oxygen (eg. Venticaire green = 60%).

Other mask designs (eg. Hudson and MC masks) will deliver higher concentrations of oxygen (40–60%), depending upon the flow rate of oxygen. The masks are all clearly labelled to indicate the oxygen concentration achieved for a given oxygen flow rate (Table 10.4).

Table 10.4: Oxygen masks, flow rates and approximate concentrations of delivered oxygen

Mask oxygen flow (litres/min)	Edingburgh (%)	MC (%)	Nasal cannulae (%)	Hudson (%)
1	25–30	–	25–30	–
2	30–35	30–50	30–35	25–38
4	35–40	40–70	32–40	35–45
6	–	55–75	–	50–60
8	–	60–75	–	55–65
10	–	65–80	–	60–75

Nasal cannulae are double cannulae which fit comfortably into the nostrils and will deliver between 25–40% oxygen depending upon the flow rate (normally 1–3 litres/minute). However, these concentrations are approximate and blood gases may need to be checked. A flow rate of 2 litres/minute will probably deliver 30% continuously, which is probably better than having oxygen delivered to the skin of the forehead which is where many masks end up (Figure 10.4). Nasal cannulae also have the advantage in not interfering with eating, drinking, wearing spectacles or talking.

c) Ensuring proper use by the patient

Keeping oxygen masks on confused or restless patients may be difficult, but it should not be forgotten that hypoxia is a common cause of restlessness and confusion. Face masks should not be allowed to sit on the patient's forehead; consideration of nasal cannulae should be made in patients who continually remove their masks. Time should be taken to explain to the patient the reason for oxygen therapy, and how it may be achieved.

Long-term oxygen therapy is sometimes used for patients with chronic respiratory failure (PaO_2 consistently less than 55 mmHg/7.5 kPa). This requires even more patient cooperation since

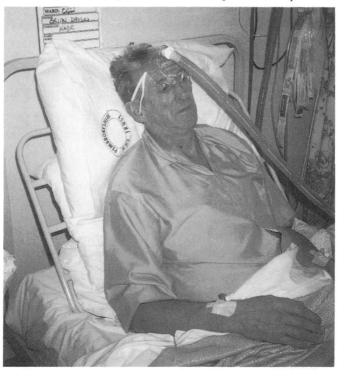

Figure 10.4 Oxygen mask on forehead

low flow-rate oxygen (1–2 litres/minute via nasal cannulae) is given for no less than 15 hours/day to prevent or reduce pulmonary hypertension, and improve prognosis.

d) Attention to humidification

Dry air or oxygen inhaled for prolonged periods stops ciliary clearing of the bronchial mucosa and promotes respiratory infection. Natural humidification only occurs with nasal respiration, so for long-term oxygen administration via mask or endotracheal tube, the oxygen must be humidified and ideally, warmed to body temperature. Bubble or surface humidifiers are preferable to nebulisers which may increase the risk of droplet infection if used long-term. Nasal cannulae and Ventimasks allow atmospheric air to mix with the oxygen which may preclude the need for humidification.

e) Preventing carbon dioxide retention

Respiratory drive is stimulated mainly by hypercapnia and to a lesser extent by hypoxia. In patients with chronic carbon dioxide retention (eg. due to chronic bronchitis), the respiratory stimulus of a high $PaCO_2$ is inoperative, so that hypoxia is the main stimulant for respiratory drive. Giving uncontrolled oxygen to these patients will abolish this drive, and they will stop breathing. There will be loss of consciousness and death ('carbon dioxide narcosis'). Oxygen therapy must therefore be controlled in order to relieve hypoxia as much as possible without abolishing the respiratory drive.

In at-risk patients requiring correction of hypoxaemia, arterial blood gases should initially be checked whilst the patient is breathing air to determine how much oxygen is likely to be tolerated. If the $PaCO_2$ is normal or low, it is safe to give over 35% oxygen, and careful monitoring is usually unnecessary. However, if the $PaCO_2$ is elevated, no more than 24% oxygen should be given initially.

After 20 minutes, the arterial blood gases should be re-checked. If the $PaCO_2$ has risen by more than 5 mmHg and the patient remains hypoxic, respiratory stimulants may be required. Higher concentrations of oxygen should not be given unless arrangements are in hand to artificially ventilate the patient.

If the $PaCO_2$ is steady, the oxygen concentration may be increased to 28%, and the blood gases repeated again after another 20 minutes. If the $PaCO_2$ is still steady, it is safe to increase the oxygen concentration to 35% if required. If however, the $PaCO_2$ has risen by more than 5 mmHg, the concentration should be returned to 24% oxygen.

Index